COMPLETE OUTDOOR SURVIVAL GUIDE

CANADIAN OUTDOOR SURVIVAL GUIDE

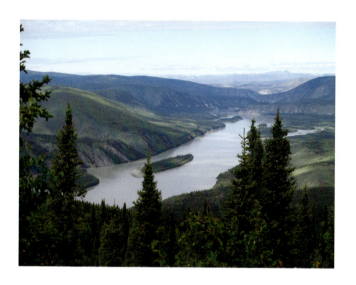

DUANE S. RADFORD

Copyright © 2021 by Lone Pine Media Productions (BC) Ltd.
Printed in China
All rights reserved. No part of this work covered by the copyrights hereon may be reproduced or used in any form or by any means—graphic, electronic or mechanical—or stored in a retrieval system or transmitted in any form by any means without the prior written permission of the publisher, except for reviewers, who may quote brief passages. Any request for photocopying, recording, taping or storage on information retrieval systems of any part of this work shall be directed in writing to the publisher.

Distributed by: Canada Book Distributors - Booklogic
www.canadabookdistributors.com
www.lonepinepublishing.com
Toll-free: 1-800-661-9017

Library and Archives Canada Cataloguing in Publication
Title: Canadian outdoor survival guide / Duane S. Radford.
Names: Radford, Duane S., 1946- author.
Identifiers: Canadiana 2021035898X | ISBN 9781551056050 (softcover)
Subjects: LCSH: Wilderness survival—Canada—Handbooks, manuals, etc.
Classification: LCC GV200.5 .R33 2022 | DDC 613.6/9—dc23Operations, issuing body IV. Title.
QK203.B7P5 2016   581.9711'1   C2016-900331-0

Editors: Ashley Bilodeau and Wendy Pirk
Layout and Production: Gregory Brown
Cover Design: Gregory Brown
Front Cover Photos: GettyImages: helivideo; Roman Barisev
Back Cover Photos: GettyImages: Ferenc Cegledi; Jupiterimages; siur
Photo Credits: *Alberta Conservation and Hunter Education Manual:* 57, 64, 94, 98, 105, 107, 108, 134, 143, 146. *GettyImages:* Akchamczuk, 121, 123; Vera Aksionava, 125; Alexandrite, 170; Pascal Alvaro, 168; Anastasiia_M, 146; anatoliy_gleb, 216; Anita, 112; anyaberkut, 80; arachi07, 200; ArgenLant, 126; ballycroy, 222; Bigmouse108, 213; bobloblaw, 171; Vladyslav Bobuskyi, 78; Ashley-Belle Burns, 76; Ines Carrara, 31; cash14, 65; Craig Chanowski, 129; Cineberg, 141; Cloudtail_the_Snow_Leopard, 192; Cobalt88, 148; cveltri, 99; DanielLacy, 145; daseaford, 71; DCrane08, 211; dndavis, 196; dobok, 137; Dr_Microbe, 116; Jozef Durok, 136; edb3_16, 95; elenabs, 149; eppicphotography, 82; Evgeny555174; Everste, 79; eyecon, 121; flyzone, 240; frontpoint, 163; Gabriele Grassl, 123; Tetiana Garkusha, 70; GeorgeBurba, 16; Sara Giacalone, 100; Aleksandr Grechanyuk, 228; gsagi, 77; gyro, 27; Hemera Technologies, 140; hive2015, 99; hobo_018, 204; Hollygraphic, 101; HSNPhotography, 58; Irina, 67; Ivan_Sabo, 180; Jeffengeloutdoors.com, 91; Joesboy, 129; jstankiewiczwitek, 124; Jupiterimages, 96; kjekol, 194; Kateryna Kolesnyk, 72; KittisakJirasittichai, 154; Krakatuk, 128; Svetlana Krayushkina, 122; Eileen Kumpf, 130; Irina Kuznetsova, 145; Elizabeth Lara, 93; lasido, 225; Tetiana Lazunova, 56; Lebazele, 44; Anhelina Lisna, 169; LOJ5407, 122; Lorerock81, 44; LucBrousseau, 212; LuCaAr, 172; Madrolly, 142; madsci, 36; MarcBruxelle, 51; marekuliasz, 61; Marius_M_Grecu, 238; mikdam, 215; Mny-Jhee, 20; MommoM_ns, 115; R Lolli Morrow, 182; MRaust, 162; Nataliia_Makarova, 105; Nataliia_Melnychuk, 25; Nazarii Neshcherenskyi, 86; Nicki1982, 98; Andrey Nikitin, 133; ninelutsk, 38; Nosyrevy, 56; Yulia Ogneva, 90; OlyaSolodenko, 128; ovanmandic, 139; PavelS, 32; Robert Pavsic, 59; PBallay, 127; Richard Phillips, 135; Photawa, 166; Photos.com, 62; photosaint, 74; piart, 13, 33, 87, 217, 241; Prostock-Studio, 153; rarrarorro, 97; REBELProductions, 197; reyj, 81; ronniechua, 161; RONSAN4D, 18; SangSanit, 69; T Schofield, 37; SeanXu, 110; Anastasia Shemetova, 41, 42, 47, 89; Devita ayu Silvianingtyas, 155; Sky_Sajjaphot, 12; Freja Solberg, 99; SolidMaks, 65; Straystone, 73; surogati, 126; Shirley Szeto, 185; Tatevrika, 68; taviphoto, 97; Kenneth Taylor, 34; Trueash, 91; TT, 73; twildlife, 179; vanVerhal, 92; Voren1, 203; vzwer, 118; Lukas Walker, 101; wanderluster, 104; warrengoldswain, 46; Wildnerdpix, 127; Евгений Харитонов, 225; yamonstro, 83; yhelfman, 195; Zakharova_Natalia, 76. *Northwest Territories Archive:* 29. *Duane Radford:* 3, 5, 6, 7, 8, 14, 15, 21, 40, 41, 48, 53, 102, 117, 145, 158, 177, 183, 220, 221, 224, 227, 229, 230, 233, 234, 236, 218, 256. *Terri Vidricaire:* 30, 176. *Wikimedia Commons:* Denelson83, 84; Cameron Hayne, 26; PeterB1903, 25; Norman Robinson, 22; Harold Wilson, 24.

DISCLAIMER:
Although the *Canadian Outdoor Survival Guide* is based on the best available information, the author and publisher do not assume any liability whatsoever for any type of accident or injury that may arise from outdoor survival techniques covered in the book.
This guide is not meant to be a "how-to" reference guide for consuming wild plants. We do not recommend experimentation by readers, and we caution that many of the plants in Canada, including some traditional medicines, are poisonous and harmful. Be aware that many plants have similar species that might be misidentified, so consumption of plants, roots and berries must be conducted with the advice of an expert.

We acknowledge the financial support of the Government of Canada.
Nous reconnaissons l'appui financier du gouvernement du Canada.

PC: 38-1

Contents

The Quitter.. 9

Acknowledgements 11

Dedication 10

Introduction 13

John Hornby: Lessons on Surviving
the Canadian North 21

SECTION I • Before You Go: Preparedness **33**

Trip Planning..35	Trekking Poles 60
Check the Weather Forecast........................35	Snowshoes..60
Understanding Local Weather Patterns......36	Flares..64
Essential Gear 38	Special Tools (Leatherman)
Survival Kits..38	and Knives 65
Pocket Survival Kit.......................................40	Axes, Hatchets and Saws 67
Vehicle Survival Kit 42	Axes..67
TRANSPORT CANADA	Hatchets..68
EMERGENCY SYMBOLS..............................43	Saws and Bow (Swede) Saws 69
Signaling Devices 45	Tents...71
Whistles..45	Tarps...73
Sprortsman's Signal Kit...............................45	Sleeping Bags and Mattresses..................... 74
ACR Firefly Rescue Lite..............................45	Technology 77
First Aid Kit...46	Communication Technology......................77
Pocket-sized First Aid Kit Components....47	Navigation Technology................................81
Commercial First Aid Kit Components......47	Maps 83
Clothing and Footwear..................................48	
Gear..58	
Backpacks..58	*(continued on next page)*
Flashlights and Headlamps 58	

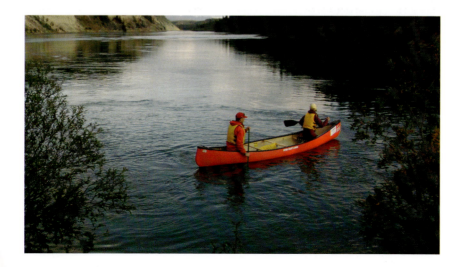

Contents

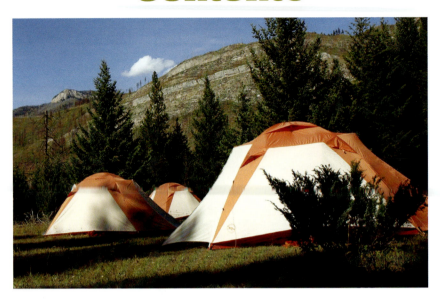

SECTION 2 • In the Field: Survival Skills 87

The "STOP" Method 88	Water 110
The "Survival Rule of Four" 89	Drinking water 110
Fire 90	Finding Water 113
Wilderness Fire Locations 93	Water Purification and Filtration 115
How to Start a Fire 94	Food: Foraging, Trapping and Fishing 120
Proper Placement of Fire 101	Foraging: Rules and Tips 120
Fire Tending 101	Safety 120
Construct a Camp Stove 101	Edible Plants 121
Shelter 102	Poisonous Plants (Wild) 127
Location 102	Nuts and Seeds 129
Keeping a Clean Campsite 103	Bird Eggs 129
Building a Shelter 104	Insects 130
Quinzee Hut 104	Porcupines and Fool Hens 131
Igloo 105	Animal Snares and Traps 133
Snow Cave 105	Fishing 135
Tarp Structures (Hammock, Wraps) 106	Survival Fishing Techniques 135
Forester's Tent 106	DIY Fishing Hooks 137
Lean-to Tent 106	Survivalist Hunting and
Lean-to Shelter 106	Fishing Legalities 137
Fallen Tree Shelter 108	Wilderness First Aid 138
Leaf Structure 108	Triage (ABCDE Rule) 140
Bough Bed 109	CPR 142
Natural Shelters and Caves 109	Frostbite: Signs, Treatment
	and Prevention 144

Contents

Hypothermia: Signs,
    Treatment and Prevention 146
Dehydration: Signs and Treatment 148
Heatstroke and Heat Exhaustion:
    Signs, Treatment and Prevention 148
Shock: Signs and Treatment 150
Wounds: Treatment and Preventing
    Infection 150
Broken Bones and Sprains 152
Head Injuries and Concussions:
    Signs and Treatment 154
Eye Injuries 155
Snake Bites 156
Insect Bites 157
Environmental Hazards 158
Preventing Wildlife Encounters 172
Backcountry Wildlife Safety 175
Navigation 205
    With a Compass 205
    Without a Compass 205
Knots 207
How to Be Found 211
Car Survival 214

SECTION 3: Specialized Outdoor Activities 217

Boat Safety and Troubleshooting 217
Legal Requirements and
    Life-Saving Appliances 218
Outboard Motorboats and
    Electric Motors 222
Off-highway Vehicle Travel 224
    Snowmobiles 224
All-terrain Vehicles (ATVs)
    and Dirt Bikes 227
Helicopter and Plane Crashes,
    Contingencies 229
Mountain Climbing 238

SECTION 4: Reflection 241

Notes 243
Appendix 248
Index 250
About the Author 256

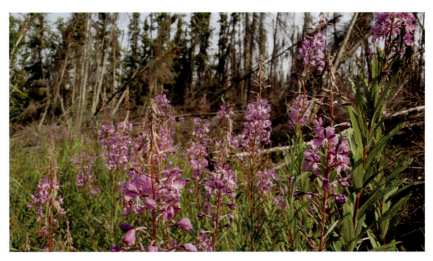

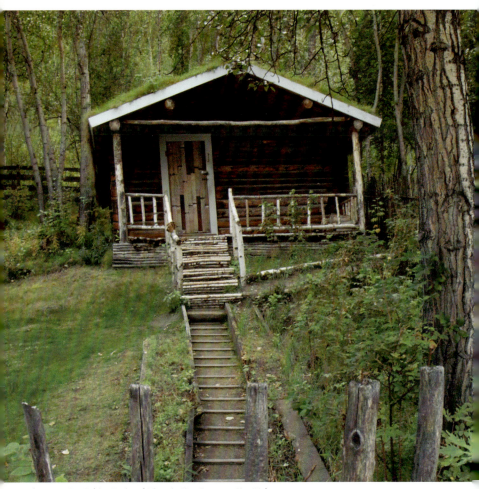
Robert Service Cabin, National Historic Site, Dawson City, Yukon.

The Quitter

When you're lost in the Wild, and you're scared as a child,
And Death looks you bang in the eye,
And you're sore as a boil, it's according to Hoyle
To cock your revolver and . . . die.
But the Code of a Man says: "Fight all you can,"
And self-dissolution is barred.
In hunger and woe, oh, it's easy to blow . . .
It's the hell-served-for-breakfast that's hard.

"You're sick of the game!" Well, now, that's a shame.
You're young and you're brave and you're bright.
"You've had a raw deal!" I know — but don't squeal,
Buck up, do your damnedest, and fight.
It's the plugging away that will win you the day,
So don't be a piker, old pard!
Just draw on your grit; it's so easy to quit:
It's the keeping-your-chin-up that's hard.

It's easy to cry that you're beaten — and die;
It's easy to crawfish and crawl;
But to fight and to fight when hope's out of sight —
Why, that's the best game of them all!
And though you come out of each grueling bout,
All broken and beaten and scarred,
Just have one more try — it's dead easy to die,
It's the keeping-on-living that's hard.

—Robert W. Service, *Rhymes of a Rolling Stone*

Dedication

I'd like to dedicate this book to my father, Samuel Owen Radford, who introduced me to camping, firearms and fishing, along with my grandfather, Albert Sapeta, and his son Carl, both of whom inspired me to be an outdoorsman with their entertaining tales of hunting, travels in the wilderness and prospecting in the far reaches of Canada.

Acknowledgements

I'd like to thank my editors, Wendy Pirk and Ashley Bilodeau, who kept me on my toes and asked the tough questions to get the content of this book right. As my University of Calgary graduate student supervisor, Professor Dr. Richard Hartland-Rowe used to say, "It shouldn't be just clear; it should be crystal clear." Wendy enjoys being outdoors and has the eye of an eagle, so she was a big help in crafting and honing the storyline along with correcting my errors. Many thanks are also due to Ashley for the changes she suggested to both the organization of the guide and suggestions for new content.

I'd also like to thank Faye Boer who represented the publisher, Shane Kennedy, and had the confidence in me to tackle this complex subject after three earlier false starts by different authors. Faye, I hope I've got it right this time around!

I turned to experts throughout the subject matter in this guide for advice and information. Jack Elliott, David O'Farrell and Larry Nagy are authorities on Indigenous history, bear self-defense and bush planes and Yukon lore, respectively. Fellow writer Don Meredith provided key information about bear sprays. Tom Bateman, Alberta's former Chief Hunter Education Officer, is the architect behind the survival kit chapter and its contents. I'd like to thank Robert (Bob) Gruszecki for providing a complimentary copy of the Alberta Conservation and Hunter Education Manual and for kindly authorizing use of the material including artwork for publication in the Canadian Outdoor Survival Guide. Thanks are also due to Terri Vidricaire, Twin Butte, Alberta, for sharing some wonderful photos of a sow grizzly bear, some of which feature her cubs.

Last, I'd like to thank my wife Adrienne with whom I've shared many outdoor trips across Canada. She provided a lot of advice and encouragement while I researched and wrote this book. Adrienne achieved the Gold Cord as a Girl Guide at a young age and has always enjoyed the outdoors. She's been there and done that and fully appreciates the challenges of Canadian outdoor adventures and just how physically demanding they can be, so she speaks from experience.

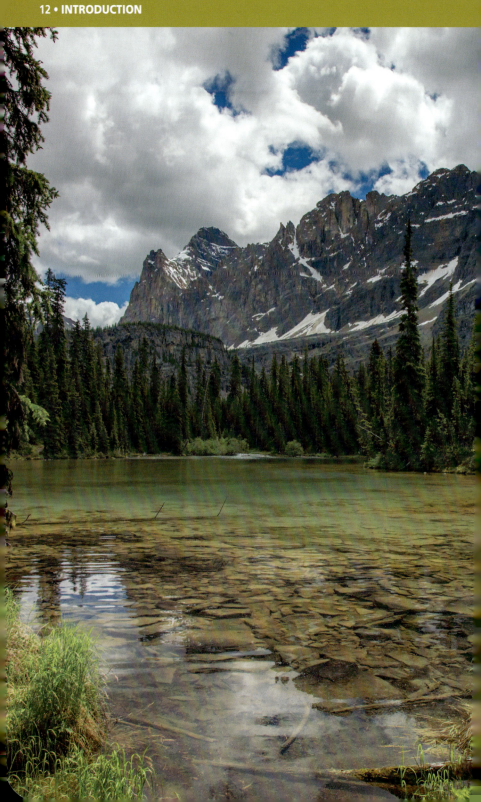

Introduction

Due to the vast tracts of inhospitable terrain and often deadly harsh weather—especially during winter—there is no country that rivals Canada.

Many historical accounts of outdoor survival in Canada are tied to the search for the Northwest Passage and expeditions to the North Pole. Others tell tales of early explorers, fur traders, prospectors, adventurers and more recently, bush pilots, all of which are full of much drama. Granted, Russia—particularly Siberia—presents similar challenges because of its geography, climate and insect pests, but it isn't as steeped in survival lore as Canada. Russian lore has it that Siberia is too vast for outsiders, too cold and unforgiving for anyone not born there and accustomed to it from birth. Perhaps the same could be said for vast parts of Canada, especially for people who spend much of their working lives in the outdoors—northern adventurers, Indigenous hunters, loggers, miners in the barren lands, trappers and commercial fishermen and women.

It is a marvel that Indigenous Peoples settled the whole of what is now Canada—the First Nations and Inuit eons ago, the Métis later on in history. Their survival story is that of a partnership of whole families and clans working as teams, with only the help of dogs before horses escaped from the Spanish conquistadors. Consequently, it is of no surprise that Indigenous Peoples guided and supported white explorers, fur traders and trappers throughout the settlement of Canada. They were skilled in the outdoors, familiar with travel routes on land and water and knew how to live off the land.

It is important that I acknowledge the Indigenous people that lived here before us. Much of what we know about survival in the Canadian wilderness was taught to us by the First Nation, Inuit and Métis peoples. Early Canadian explorers depended on them to secure food and to travel in unknown country by living off the land during their travels.

Some Canadian survival stories are of such epic proportions as the expedition when Captain Sir John Franklin was compelled to abandon his doomed ships, *Erebus* and *Terror*, in April 1848 and begin a southerly trip toward civilization where all hands perished. In the period preceding and following the First World War, the legends of English traveler John Hornby in the Arctic and subarctic are equally astonishing. (Some of Hornby's stories will be covered in a separate chapter because they are so germane to this book.) There is the more recent, tragic tale of Martin Hartwell, who in 1972 survived an Arctic medivac crash—

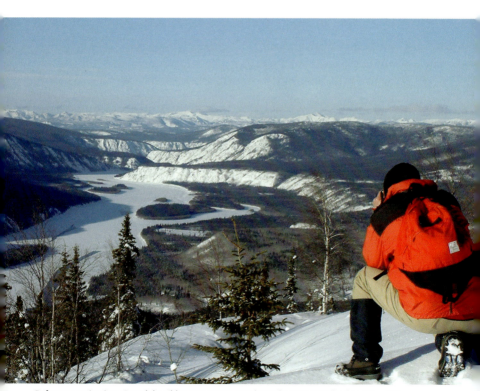

Before venturing into Canada's wilderness, ensure you have the necessary backcountry skills.

INTRODUCTION • 15

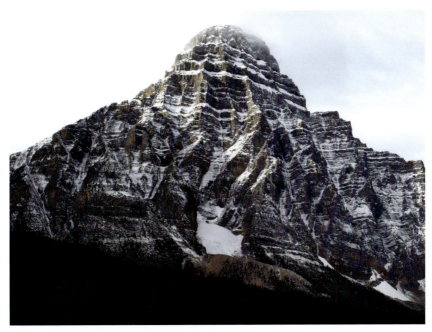

Mountain climbers should be prepared for avalanches.

which killed two passengers, while another died later—for 31 days in the barren lands of the Northwest Territories under unspeakably brutal weather conditions. I will draw on circumstances tied to these historical events where appropriate to illustrate what can go wrong and hopefully help readers avoid an unfavorable ending on their own trips in the wilds of Canada.

The salient message in a brochure *Into the Yukon Wilderness* bears repeating here: Before venturing into Canada's wilderness, ensure you have the necessary backcountry skills. If you don't have these skills, then you're putting yourself and other members of your party at risk. Before starting your trip, take a course on outdoor recreation or survival skills, or have an experienced friend mentor you. Begin with short, day trips before going on longer, overnight trips in the backcountry. Unlike early explorers and trappers, you need a licence to hunt and fish and can only do so during open seasons, subject to the ordinances in place, so don't expect to live off the land. To illustrate this point, the Canadian government mandated that prospectors venturing into the Yukon during the Klondike goldrush be provisioned with at least one ton of supplies so they would be adequately provisioned to ward off mass starvation.

Another key message is that anybody can get caught in a hazardous situation; so, as the Boy Scout and

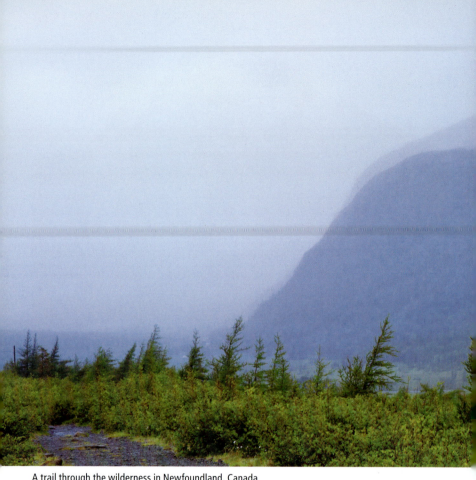

A trail through the wilderness in Newfoundland, Canada

Girl Guide mottos state, "Be prepared." By this motto, "scouts" and "guides" are ready to cope with anything that might come their way.

Over a coffee at Awesome Lake, my Labrador fishing guide, Orville Caddy, chuckled. "Be prepared for the worst… It could rain, it could snow, it could do just about everything. The hardest thing up here is the wind we've had this past 15 days. It blowed every single day, really hard. I'm talking about at least 25 or 30 mile an hour wind. That's what you got to expect. You got to expect the worst. And if it's pretty, you got it made… that's a bonus."

On the way home, over a beer in St. John's, Newfoundland, one of the locals and I got to talking. "In Labrador, you can have all four seasons in one day," he said with a shrug. This is also a favourite saying among ranchers in Alberta where the

INTRODUCTION • 17

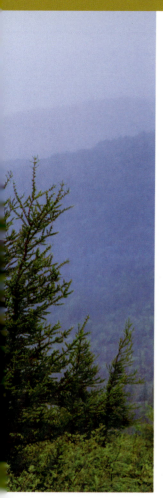

weather can be fickle, especially in the foothills of the Rocky Mountains. Outdoorspeople should take a page from local knowledge: plan for the best and prepare for the worst. I've had some brushes with death of my own, including a terrifying helicopter crash in 1978 near Three Lakes Ridge on the Alberta Rockies High Rock Range that I'll elaborate on in the section Helicopter and Plane Crashes and Contingencies (p. 231) as a teachable event, among other trips I've made in bush planes and helicopters that could have ended badly. You will find anecdotal stories sprinkled throughout the book to highlight my experience in the Canadian outdoors and emphasize why the lessons in this book should be taken seriously.

There are no comprehensive national records regarding outdoor related deaths in Canada, although some recent information on the leading causes provides enough information to put matters into perspective. Drownings, helicopter and small aircraft accidents, overexposure, avalanches and bear attacks are among the leading causes of death in the outdoors. In the most recent five-year period (2010–2014) reported, an average of 464 people drowned in Canada each year, down slightly from an average of 489 per year in

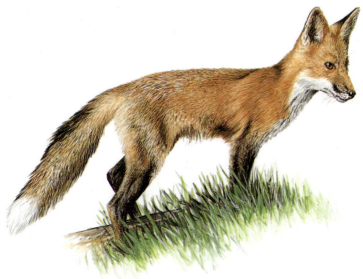

2005–2009. Canadian-registered aircraft, excluding ultralights, were reported in 173 accidents in 2018 (191 including the 18 accidents involving ultralights). This is lower than the 208 accidents reported in 2017 and 25 percent below the annual average of 230 accidents over the preceding 10 years. Winter temperature combined with wind chill can cause severe injuries and even death. More than 80 people die each year in Canada from over-exposure to the cold, and there is an average of 14 avalanche-related deaths in Canada every year, most occurring in British Columbia and western Alberta. Bear encounters

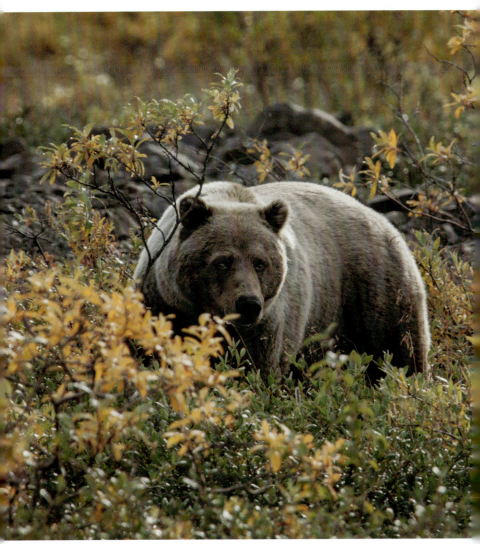

Grizzly bear forages in dwarf willow

Before venturing into Canada's wilderness, ensure you have the necessary backcountry skills. If you don't have these skills, you're putting yourself and other members of your party at risk.

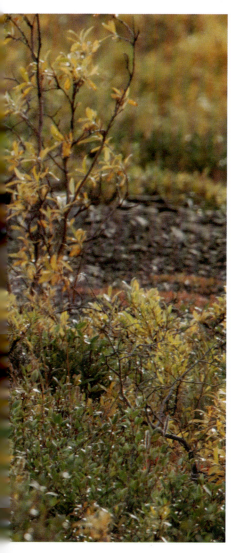

are increasing in Canada and worldwide as more people recreate in bear country and as bear numbers increase in western provinces due to closed hunting seasons on grizzly bears. Between 1997 and 2017, 25 fatal black bear attacks have occurred in North America. In Canada, six of these deaths occurred in British Columbia and three in Quebec. In my opinion, the number of bear attacks in Canada is likely underreported, an opinion that is shared by many experienced outdoorspeople.

The Canadian wilderness is a unique outdoor environment. As such, this is a stand-alone book about survival in the Canadian wild, not the jungles of Asia, Africa and South America or the world's deserts, where travel is challenging because of overexposure to the heat, a lack of water or deadly diseases, not to mention dangerous animals such as alligators, crocodiles and poisonous snakes and constrictors.

Notwithstanding this sobering prelude, this guidebook is intended to be a useful learning and reference tool for novices who go out for a hike and run into trouble and even for

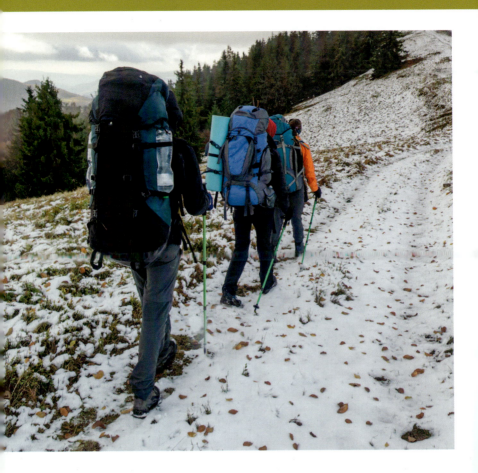

more experienced outdoorspeople who journey into Canada's wilderness where danger lurks. The content is both practical and relevant. It is not intended to frighten people from venturing outdoors, but rather offer ways to make such trips safe and rewarding. Covering everything from how to prepare for a trip to what to do during a situation gone wrong where your life might be at stake, this is the one book that you should read and perhaps take with you just in case something goes wrong. Help is often just around the corner if disaster strikes—Canada has outstanding search and rescue capabilities operated by the military, Royal Canadian Mounted Police, volunteer organizations, local police forces and federal and provincial park authorities—but that still doesn't negate the need for outdoor survival skills.

Author Note: I will switch from English to metric units of measurement throughout the book, as would be the custom for the particular chapter contents.

John Hornby: Lessons on Surviving the Canadian North

For those whose adventures take them North of Sixty—the geographic parallel that separates Yukon, Northwest Territories and Nunavut from the southern provinces, it's instructive to reflect on at least some of John Hornby's key travels described in *The Legend of John Hornby* by George Whalley (1962). The enormity of the expanse of rugged mountains, bush and barren lands, characteristic of northern Canada, cannot be appreciated or comprehended until a person has traveled extensively in these wilderness areas.

Hornby suffered through and survived just about every possible misadventure that's relevant to outdoor survival, so it's only fitting that a chapter in this book be devoted to his experiences because they are still relevant. Game laws, however, have changed, and living off the land is now subject to fishing and hunting regulations. Trapping is also regulated and subject to registered traplines on Crown land and/or by landowner permission-only on private land. Strictly speaking, it's not feasible for settlers "to live off the land" anymore (throughout the course of a year), although many Indigenous

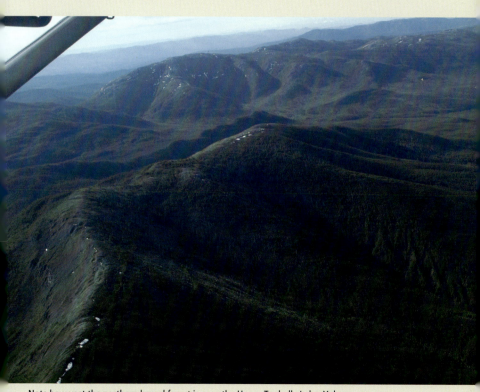

Note how vast the northern boreal forest is near the Upper Toobally Lake, Yukon.

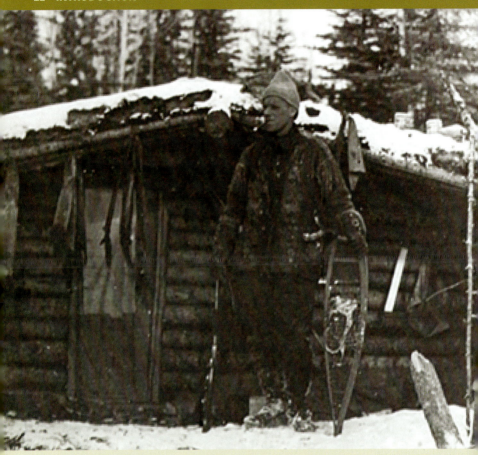

John Hornby in front of one of his remote trapping cabins

Peoples in Canada still do so, largely leading a subsistence lifestyle. It is also illegal to trap unless it is in accordance with trapping regulations. Hornby was not subject to these regulations. (Neither was R.M. Patterson, whose exploits in the Nahanni River, Northwest Territories, are referenced in his book: *The Dangerous River*.)

Even though he was a remarkable, tough as nails, individual, Hornby's luck eventually ran out, and he met his demise because of some critical errors in judgement. He was a fascinating person, despite being characterized by Whalley as being "irreverent" at times and having "muddling, confused and ill-directed ways." In a matter of just a few years, his reputation evolved to become that of a legendary figure in the laurels of bushcraft, as he quickly gained experience in dealing with natural hazards and travel in the bush.

Hornby first came to Canada from England in 1904 at age 23 for adventure from all accounts. He had many close calls with death, and the final

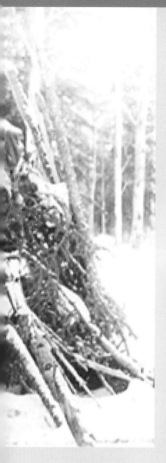

By all accounts, he had extraordinary athletic qualities that would greatly surpass those of most outdoorspeople. He claimed that all the gear he needed "even for journeys of indefinite duration" in the bush was a rifle, a bag of flour and a fish net.

chapter in his life happened "when the caribou didn't come" during a trip where just about everything that could go wrong did go wrong. Hornby was an extraordinary frontier's man by any standard, a trail blazer who seemingly had no quit. While small in stature, weighing only about 100 pounds and standing around 5 feet 4 inches tall, he was incredibly strong and tough. Hornby was known to carry a load of 125 pounds of caribou meat a short distance into camp—no small feat. He was not regarded as a particularly good rifleman, though there's a story about him killing four caribou with four shots on the Casba (Lochhart) River with a companion's rifle with open sights, also no small feat.

As examples of feats of his endurance, lore has it that while living near Edmonton, Alberta, Hornby made a 100-mile run to Athabasca Landing on the Athabasca River in twenty-four hours, as well as a 50-mile run beside a horse to Lac Ste Anne, east of Edmonton. By all accounts, he had extraordinary athletic qualities that would greatly surpass those of most outdoorspeople. He claimed that all the gear he needed "even for journeys of indefinite duration" in the bush was a rifle, a bag of flour and a fish net. This is a lesson that should not be lost on outdoors folks, to a degree: travel light and take only what you need to survive in Canada's outdoors, but make sure you have everything you need. This misgiving was the demise of over-burdened men of the Franklin expedition who were badly weighed down by useless items they ferried along their escape route.

There is a telling notation in Hornby's diary during the winter of 1920-21 when he lived in isolation in a small six by eight-foot cabin at

Fort Reliance. "At times this life appears strange: I never see anyone, no longer have anything to read, and my pencil is too small to permit me to do much writing. It is not surprising that men go mad. I have not gone completely native yet, but unquestionably my mind has become somewhat vacant for there is nothing to sharpen the intellect. The effect of this is felt in civilization—I find it difficult to grasp what people say." (Regarding the reference to going "native", this is a long-standing undeserved denigration of Indigenous Peoples by some white settlers who wrongly assume that their lifestyle is somehow superior to that of Indigenous Peoples.)

Outdoor survival skills must address being able to cope with deprivation and isolation if a person finds themselves alone or lost in the wilderness. There is no simple solution to this issue of concern because contact with other people is important to keep one's spirits well and to maintain a positive outlook. Too much solitude can be a death sentence for all but the most optimistic people.

After spending another grim winter at Reliance without much to show for it, Hornby went out to Edmonton in the summer of 1922, later staying on in northeastern Alberta. According to reports, Hornby "was commencing to go to pieces now" and hardship "was

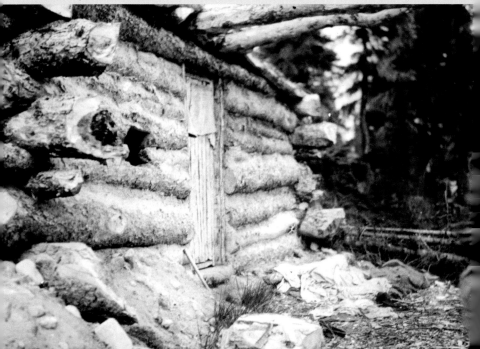

John Hornby's cabin in 1929

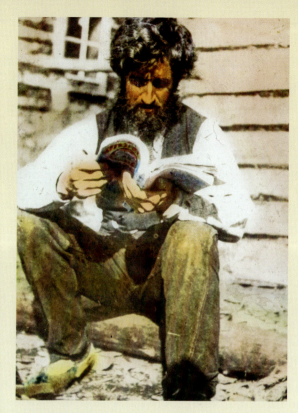

John Hornby at Fort Resolution, N.W.T., 1924

There is no room for being reckless in the bush when help can be so far away.

commencing to tell on his fortitude." He was also apparently suffering from an obsession that he could and must live off the land and didn't take sufficient flour and staple foods, a tiding that would ultimately lead to his undoing. Records of what he actually did during this time are rather spotty, but tales indicated he was becoming foolhardy and likely overestimating his abilities. In my research of stories related to Canadian outdoor survival skills, there's a recurring theme that people who perished often displayed signs of being overconfident and failing to follow a precautionary approach when in dangerous situations. There is no room for being reckless in the bush when help can be so far away.

The final chapter of Whalley's book about John Hornby is appropriately called "The Last Journey 1926-7." The chapter chronicles a sad tale that begins with a commentary on the Northern

Outdoor survival skills must address being able to cope with deprivation and isolation if a person finds themselves alone or lost in the wilderness.

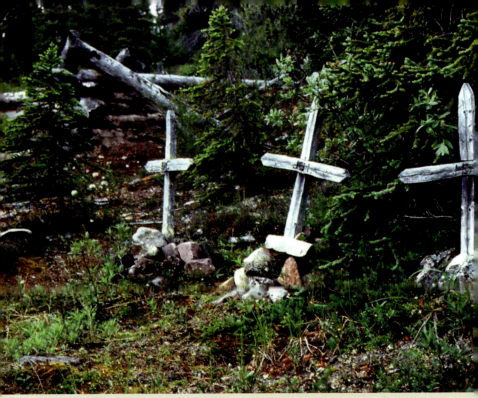

John Hornby's cabin on the Thelon River

Alberta Railway that runs through the bush and muskeg north of Edmonton to Waterways, forming a short cut to the northerly flowing Athabasca River, a line that was completed in 1916. The end of the line was at Waterways, near Fort McMurray.

I travelled overnight on this railway in 1965 when there was still no all-season road—only a winter road—into Fort McMurray. I can attest to its remarkable construction over such challenging terrain. At times it moved at a snail's pace so as not to become dislodged from the tracks.

Hornby was venturing to the Northwest Territories once again, this time with an Englishman, his cousin Edgar Christian, and another young Englishman, Harold Adlard, who was an acquaintance of Hornby. Christian's father felt the trip "would give the boy something to build his life on." It is hard looking back to fathom the ignorance and overconfidence of some people of the day. Their destination was the barren grounds along the Thelon River east of Great Slave Lake where Hornby thought trapping would be good. To their knowledge, no white man had ever trapped there before. Interestingly, there is an account of how they dealt with mosquitos—ubiquitous to the north and which they considered "their worst enemy"—by sitting in the smudge of a campfire. They also report using a mosquito net to ward off mosquitos, which affected Christian in that his ankles were swollen so badly he couldn't walk. There are other notations in notes left by Hornby regarding "flies bad," a testament to this persistent plague of the north. There's also a reference to eating bannock along with pemmican. Bannock has long been a staple in the diets of people who live in the bush for extended periods of time. I've eaten bannock prepared by Dene Peoples and Inuit women who did not seem to make it with the same ingredients or the same way, but I found it both filling and nourishing.

When they reached Reliance, Hornby declined to purchase more provisions at a local trading post. All the trappers he encountered there and along the way said the same thing—that he had very little provisions and no dogs. Hornby had by this time developed an aversion to dogs, which required a lot of upkeep and dog food to keep on the trail. Nobody saw any members of Hornby's party alive after they departed Reliance for the Thelon River to the site 350 miles away that Hornby had in mind. There is no written record of their journey into the Thelon River.

Much of the content of Whalley's book about Hornby's travels came from Hornby's diaries and personal correspondence. However, some information about the trip came from two notes he left in rock cairns in conspicuous

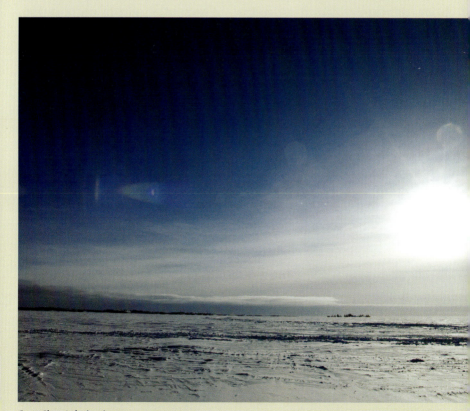

Great Slave Lake in winter

places so that they would be found by other parties en route to the Thelon River. One thing that is clear from the notes, later found by a party of prospectors, is that they were travelling so slowly there was a grave danger they would miss the southward caribou migration. Based on entries to Edgar Christian's diary it appears they were ready to move into a 14-foot square log cabin in mid-October, but by this time most of the caribou had left the area. Whalley notes that by late November "they were not starving; but they had defied the immemorial custom of the North in failing to lay in plenty of caribou in September." They had hoped to find caribou and musk ox in the area (the latter protected by government regulations) but this did not materialize. There were, however, quite a few ptarmigans around their cabin, which they tried to catch in a net with meagre results. They did shoot some from time to time with high powered rifles. If they had brought a shotgun it's likely they could have survived by living off ptarmigans.

By December they had made plans to ration what little food they had left and were down to eating what furbearers they caught in traps—foxes, hares and wolverine. They continued to set a net in the Thelon River with little to show for their efforts. By Christmas Eve, the temperature had plummeted to -45°C with very little fresh meat to eat. The obvious was happening as winter set in. They craved and needed calories that were not available. The cold became unbearable as their failure to kill caribou "deprived them of skin clothes against the winter weather," wrote Whalley. They managed to shoot one bull caribou in January, but it was eaten within a few days.

I find this report hard to believe as there should have been about 75 pounds of meat. Both Hornby and Adlard suffered from frostbite to their hands and face while Christian could scarcely endure the cold outside at all. Conditions continued to worsen over the winter and by March were grim. They were down to eating boiled hides. If they had dogs, they could have travelled at large to hunt caribou and musk ox or made a retreat to Reliance for help, which they could have reached in a week or ten days by dog sled. The men were all emaciated by the end of March. The end was near. On April 10, 1927 Hornby wrote his will before passing away in his sleep on April 17th, followed by Adlard on May 4th. On what may have been June 2nd Christian died inside their cabin after putting the party's documents inside the stove with a note written on a piece of paper on top saying: "WHO [EVER COMES HERE] LOOK IN STOVE."

On July 21, 1927, a group of four prospectors led by H.S. Wilson discovered Hornby's cabin, finding two corpses outside and a third corpse on a bed inside. Wilson noted, "Bodies apparently those of J. Hornby & his two nephews." Wilson's party departed without touching anything or burying the bodies, leaving it to the authorities to investigate what happened. It wasn't until the following year that a Royal Canadian Mounted Police patrol reached the cabin and dealt with the grim situation of the two corpses outside the cabin, practically skeletons by this point. They found various papers and the remains of Christian's body and his diary inside the stove, so as to establish the dates and causes of death. The police decided that an inquest was not necessary. The bodies were buried, the crosses marked with their initials and the cabin tidied as best possible before the patrol departed for Reliance, and so ended the final chapter in the life of John Hornby, who died of starvation at age 47.

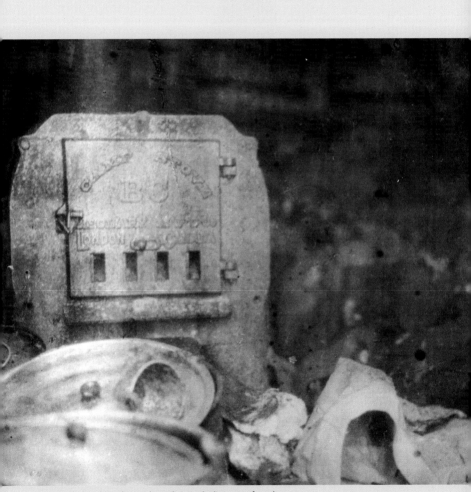

Stove in Hornby's cabin where Edgar Christian's diary was found

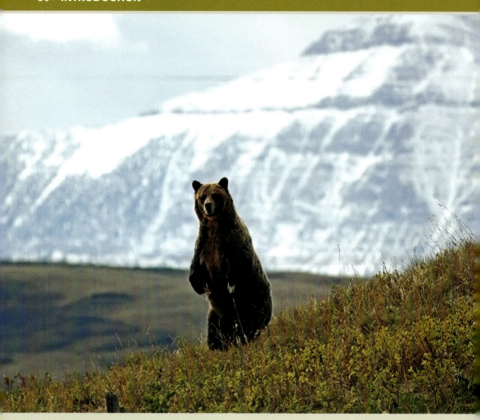

Lessons Learned

There are many morals related to the saga of John Hornby, who travelled for about 24 years in some of the most unhospitable areas of Canada and had several brushes with death before his luck finally ran out. Despite being a man of extraordinary strength and stamina, he met his demise largely because he was improperly provisioned on his final journey. What lessons can we learn from his time in the wilderness of Canada's far north?

The ensuing chapters of this book will illustrate survival techniques that date back to Hornby's era as well as explore outdoor survival techniques in the modern era. Hornby did not have topographic maps to guide him, often only hand sketches provided by other adventurers and fur traders, some of which were loaded with errors. He did not know how to swim; it's remarkable that he didn't drown considering how much time he spent on treacherous, turbulent rivers and the waters of often dangerous, immense lakes.

Hornby had some close encounters with barren ground grizzly bears, which he had to shoot in self-defence, a testament to the threats they pose. It is of paramount importance that today's travelers be prepared for encounters with black bears, grizzly bears and polar bears in Canada's wilderness. If you doubt this assertion, several chapters in Ken Bailey's book *No Place Like Home* (2019) vividly illustrate what might happen with all three species, especially while hunting in remote areas.

Based on Hornby's journal, it appears that he and his companions were not properly clothed for the brutal weather they encountered on the barrens in his final journey and suffered frostbite and probably hypothermia. Nowadays, there is no excuse for not being prepared for long periods of freezing weather in Canada.

It's important for outdoorspeople to get in top shape before they venture into the outdoors on extended trips in the back country. From all accounts, Hornby was in remarkable physical condition, which probably saved his life on many occasions. Regardless, he did become ill and incapacitated, which speaks to the need for first aid training and state-of-the-art first aid kits for adventurers. Further, Hornby often spoke of the ill effects of ubiquitous mosquitoes and black flies in the Northwest Territories, which can drive people crazy and inflame their limbs after being bitten numerous times. You must have insect repellent and proper clothing to contend with them.

Don't travel alone. Traveling solo is a dangerous practice. Hornby's companions saved him on more than one occasion when he became ill. Be sure to have a plan that includes leaving instructions with reliable authorities in case a mishap occurs. Hornby did not leave a detailed plan on his final journey, and this put authorities who searched for him in danger. It also made this search all the more difficult and time consuming before his remains and those of his companions were eventually discovered.

Black fly

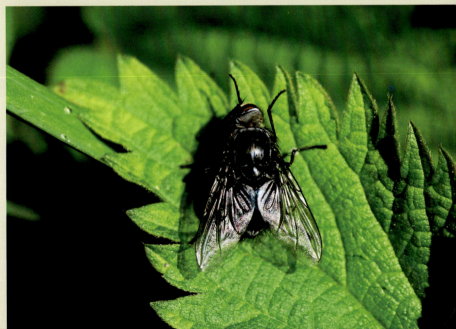

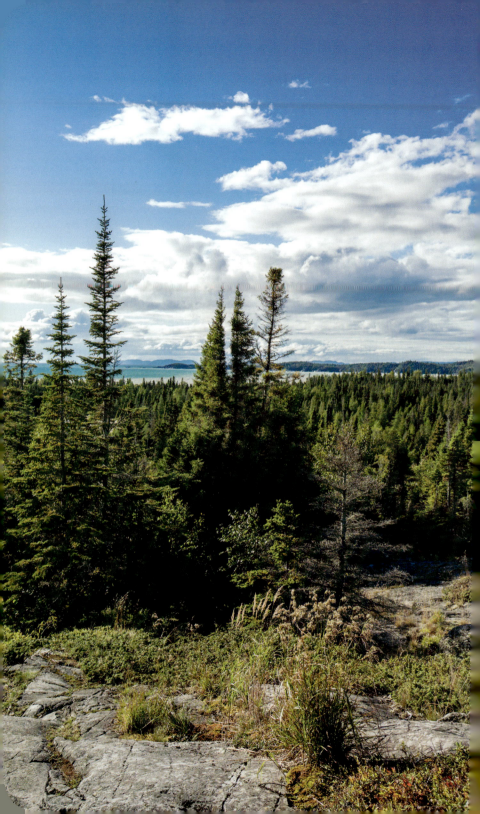

SECTION 1
Before You Go: Preparedness

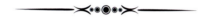

The wilderness offers no guarantees.

This book was written during the Covid-19 pandemic that started in Canada in March 2020. The pandemic reinforced the old cliché, "You should travel while you still can," in more ways than one, not only related to a person's health, as the entire country was gripped in a nationwide lockdown over the course of several months. Once the lockdown was relaxed, people in my home province of Alberta flocked to the outdoors in unparalleled numbers never seen before in my lifetime. Headlines in local newspapers soon started to report on all manner of outdoor accidents—deaths by drowning, falls on mountain trails, etc.—quite likely by people who did not have much experience in the outdoors and were not properly prepared. Regrettably, some of the casualties were new Canadians who were not familiar with wilderness hazards. Many of them drowned in backcountry rivers. However, there were lots of Canadian nationals who also met their demise while boating and hiking, many of whom were young people. There were also reports of folks being mauled by cougars and bears in British Columbia and Saskatchewan, testament to the importance of always being vigilant around wild animals.

While the Canadian wilderness is a wonderful place to visit, it is also dangerous, so wilderness travel

Pukaskwa National Park, Ontario

Before venturing into Canada's wilderness, "ensure you have the necessary backcountry skills."

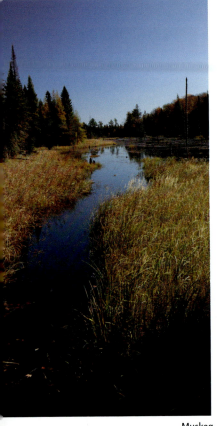
Muskeg

should never be taken lightly. You cannot expect the weather to be good in the wilderness. Often it rains for days on end with strong, chilling winds that can cause hypothermia, and it is not unusual for water buckets to freeze over in the Alberta Rockies, even in the middle of summer. If you do not have adequate outdoor apparel, your time might well be miserable. Water is usually available throughout most of Canada, but not all of it is potable, especially in areas of muskeg whose waters can make some people sick. Even what look to be safe streams may be contaminated with bacteria. You should always purify water.

Don't take anything for granted before you leave home, and make sure you have a checklist of essential items such as water, enough food to last the trip with some in reserve, warm clothing, a shelter if you're going to be spending time overnight and a contingency plan in case something goes wrong. Even in areas that have established trails and backcountry shelters, people can and do get lost and not all stories have a happy ending. Preparedness and practiced outdoor survival skills are essential to fun and safe outdoor adventures.

Preparedness and practiced outdoor survival skills are essential to fun and safe outdoor adventures.

Trip Planning

Outdoor travelers should share their daily schedule with their loved ones so if they don't return when expected, the proper authorities can be alerted to start a search for them.

It is only common sense that, regardless of where you are hiking, you tell a family member, friend or neighbour about your plans. While accidents or misadventures are rare, tell them where you're going and when you plan to return.

Research the area you plan to travel in and tell someone where you are going.

Check the Weather Forecast

When it comes to local hiking, I always check online weather forecasts before I head outdoors. What is the temperature going to be, is there a chance of rain, what about winds? The weather report is your guide to what kind of apparel you should wear during a hike and any extra items you might need in case of contingencies.

If you are not an outdoor adventurer, there is no better time to start than during the summer. In Canada, summer days are long, temperatures are comfortable and the weather is usually ideal to spend time in the outdoors. If you haven't done any hiking, start small and work your way up to longer hikes. Choose the right trail for your level of fitness to begin with. It can be challenging for beginners to get their bearings. Familiarize yourself with the trails by studying a map before you set out so you know where you're going.

Job number one is always to get a map that illustrates the route you plan to hike, whether it's an established trail or cross-country.

Always check online weather forecasts before heading outdoors.

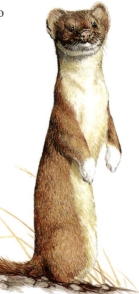

Understanding Local Weather Patterns

If you aren't familiar with the area where you intend to travel, you should research local weather patterns early in the planning stages well

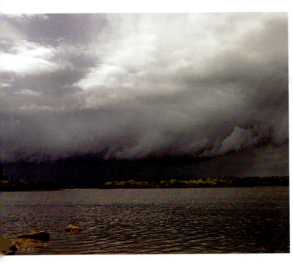

before your trip. Certain parts of Canada are well known for peculiar, long-established weather patterns. The Coast Mountain Range in British Columbia is characterized by heavy precipitation during the winter. They form a major mountain range in the *Pacific Coast Ranges* of western North America, extending from southwestern Yukon through the Alaska Panhandle and virtually all of the coast of British Columbia south to the Fraser River. Terrace, near the mid-part of the Coast Range, receives 40+ inches of rain annually, on average. Many Coast Mountain Range streams have braided channels because there are so many floods, and, consequently, it is dangerous to camp near their banks. The foothills of southwestern Alberta from Calgary down to the United States border experience powerful chinook winds, sometimes reaching near-hurricane speed. The Blackfoot people call this wind *Snow Eater* because it can swallow up snow overnight when temperatures might go from −20°C to 10°C within 24 hours. Gale-force winds often mark Canada's western Arctic, often for several days in a row or longer. It is virtually impossible for planes to fly under these circumstances. Likewise, this part of the Arctic can be subject to heavy fog banks making flights unsafe, grounding all aircraft for days on end. Winter blizzards can last for long periods of time in the barren grounds. Heavy precipitation can fall in most parts of Newfoundland and Labrador for days on end. Once, while I was staying at Awesome Lake, Labrador, it had rained so much that the water level in the lake came up by almost 2 feet.

Strait of Georgia, British Columbia

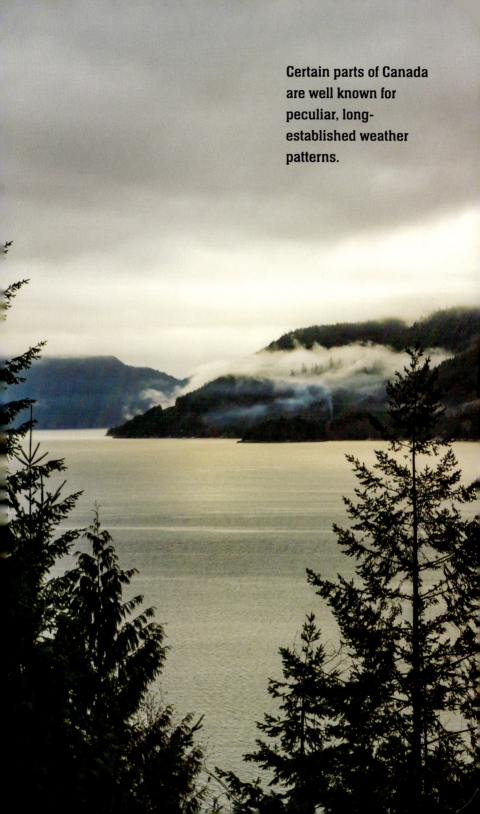

Certain parts of Canada are well known for peculiar, long-established weather patterns.

Essential Gear

Survival Kits

A survival kit could mean the difference between life and death.

The best survival kit is small and compact enough to be carried in a pocket or your jacket. Outdoorspeople should never get complacent about wilderness survival and never assume that they won't be caught in a situation where they need a survival kit.

Depending on the nature of your travels in the backcountry, you may wish to customize a personal kit based on your needs. Remember, however, that if your kit is too large, it may be impractical to carry it and could even become a hindrance when escaping a hazardous situation. If your travels are such that you don't think you need to carry a kit on your person, you could put the contents in a larger, plastic or metal water bottle with a large lid so the contents can fit into it easily.

I have had several close calls when in the bush, some on lakes and rivers when I worked in northern Alberta, and the worst being a terrifying helicopter crash on the High Rock Range in Alberta's Rockies. Now, whenever I am travelling in remote

Breaking Fast
Health care professionals will provide advice on "breaking fast" if you haven't eaten any food for a long period of time. Avoid breaking your fast with a meal that is high in carbohydrates and sugar. Instead, you should stick to low-carb, high-fat meals. As well, be sure to stay hydrated during your fast.

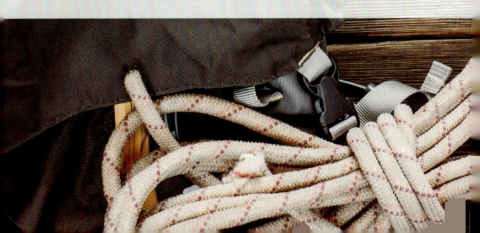

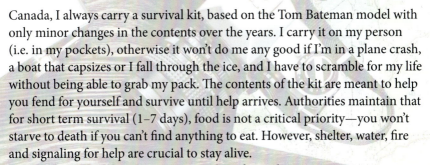

Canada, I always carry a survival kit, based on the Tom Bateman model with only minor changes in the contents over the years. I carry it on my person (i.e. in my pockets), otherwise it won't do me any good if I'm in a plane crash, a boat that capsizes or I fall through the ice, and I have to scramble for my life without being able to grab my pack. The contents of the kit are meant to help you fend for yourself and survive until help arrives. Authorities maintain that for short term survival (1–7 days), food is not a critical priority—you won't starve to death if you can't find anything to eat. However, shelter, water, fire and signaling for help are crucial to stay alive.

The contents of the Bateman Survival Kit fit inside a small, metal tobacco can (1 x 3.25 x 4.5 inches in size) that is sealed with Johnson & Johnson First Aid waterproof adhesive tape. In a pinch, you can empty the tobacco can and use it to heat water to make yourself some broth or tea and use it for cooking. The adhesive tape keeps the contents dry if you go in the water or get caught in the rain. The tape can also be used, if necessary, for medical purposes.

You must be familiar with the contents in your survival kit and understand how to use them before you leave home.

You must be familiar with the contents in your survival kit and understand how to use them before you leave home. The needles and thread can be used to stitch cuts and wounds as well as mend clothing. Cuts to the bone will not heal without stitches. Your best bet to obtain food in the short term is by fishing and catching small game with snares. The fishing lures are some of Canada's top producers and all have a history of go-to terminal tackle, although you may have others you prefer. Make sure your flies are ideal for the area you are travelling in. Some snare wire will come in handy to catch hares that are common throughout Canada. The rest of the contents are standard items for wilderness survival in Canada.

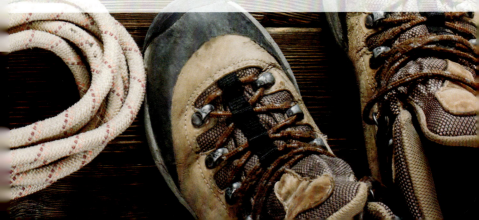

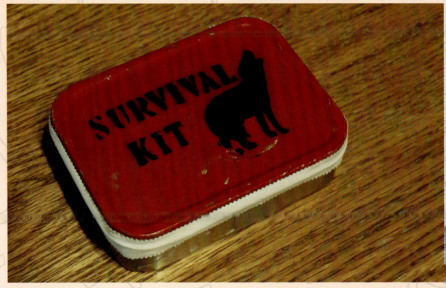

A customized survival kit can fit into a tobacco can

Pocket Survival Kit

Below is a list of the contents in my survival kit with a brief explanation of their purpose. Study the layout of the contents in the survival kit photo (p. 41), which fit best positioned a certain way.

- 2–3 feet of snare wire (coiled so that it will fit snuggly on the inside of the lid), to catch rabbits for example Several finishing nails (multi-purpose) for fastening snare wire to trees, etc.
- ~30 feet monofilament fishing line (coiled so that it will fit inside the snare wire when it is inside the lid) that can be tied to a willow, for example, to catch different species of fish
- needles and silk or surgical thread
- some bandages for small scrapes and bruises
- "Old Timer" 3-bladed pocketknife (make sure the blades are sharpened), a reliable and trusty knife
- Handheld "ERMA SG67E" signal flare and red flares (distress) to signal aircraft
- Large safety pin with half a dozen smaller safety pins for contingencies

- Waterproof matches (sealed in plastic wrap to stop them from abrading)

- "Sparking Insert Shaving Blade," cotton balls and box cutter blade to strike against the blade in an angled, downward motion to create sparks and ignite the cotton ball to start a fire

- Selection of fishing lures (e.g., miniature Len Thompson, Mepps and Panther Martin lures; several popular wet flies and streamers and several small fishing hooks)

- Selection of small rubber core twist lock lead sinkers to get a hook down in a lake

- "Rescue Flash Signal Mirror" (commercial grade) to reflect sunlight and signal aircraft

- Teabags, beef stock, salt

- Paper to keep notes and a small pencil to write with

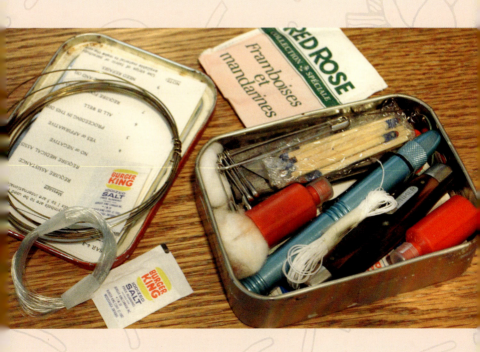

Vehicle Survival Kit

In case of a breakdown, it is a good idea to have an emergency kit in your vehicle. The following is a list of items that the Canadian Automobile Association recommends including in your vehicle's emergency kit:

- Flashlight (preferably hand crank-type because batteries don't last long in extreme cold)
- Reflective safety triangles or flares
- Small first-aid kit
- Snow brush and scraper
- Traction aids
- Small shovel with long handle
- Bag of abrasive material: sand, kitty litter (avoid road salt, which can cause your vehicle to rust)
- Plenty of windshield washer fluid
- Booster cables
- Gas-line antifreeze
- Lock de-icer (in extreme cold, keep it with you, rather than in your vehicle)
- Paper towels
- Small tool kit (screwdriver, pliers, etc.)
- Extra fuses (for the vehicle's electrical system)
- Warm blanket
- Extra socks, boots and gloves
- Hand and foot warmers
- Bottles of water
- Granola bars
- I would also add some wax candles along with a deep tin and matches to the above list to ward off the cold should you become stranded and have to remain inside a vehicle until help arrives.

Remember: Hope for the best and prepare for the worst.

Is your vehicle equipped with all the gear you might need to operate under adverse weather conditions?

Do you have a tow rope and an extension cord for your block heater, winter survival gear for you and your companions in the event of an emergency?

TRANSPORT CANADA EMERGENCY SYMBOLS

Transport Canada official message "code symbol" index inside the lid of the survival kit, to be used to communicate with aircraft when an emergency exists (see sidebar). The symbols "V" and "X" are the most important and should be stamped in the snow or laid out with evergreen branches large enough to be seen from the air.

Message	Code Symbol
REQUIRE ASSISTANCE	V
REQUIRE MEDICAL ASSISTANCE	X
NO or NEGATIVE	N
YES or AFFIRMATIVE	Y
PROCEEDING IN THIS DIRECTION	→
ALL IS WELL	LL
REQUIRE FOOD & WATER	F
REQUIRE FUEL AND OIL	L
NEED REPAIRS	W

High-energy Snacks

High-energy snacks are foods that are high in calories such as granola bars or trail mix. Bringing high-energy snacks on a trip is really a matter of personal choice. In my case, I usually carry them, but only use them in a pinch, whereas others might use them on a more regular basis. I don't eat high-energy snacks on a regular basis when hiking, hunting or fishing, only if I feel I need an energy boost. Your best bet is to start the day with healthy breakfast so you don't experience an energy sag. Based on my experience, I also suggest having a larger meal at lunch than at dinner if you're really exerting yourself outdoors, though this is only possible if you are on a planned trip. If you are in an emergency situation where you don't have a camp to go back to, high-energy snacks in your survival kit can be very helpful to keep you nourished until you are found. Use your common sense and by all means pack high-energy bars in case of emergencies.

Matches and Lighters

I prefer matches that are both waterproof and windproof. If you are using old-fashioned, strike anywhere matches, keep them in a waterproof container so they stay dry. Over time, the old-fashioned, strike anywhere match heads will deteriorate, so make sure they're useable before your trip.

While it may be hard to believe, the classic Zippo, fuel-operated (butane) and windproof lighter still remains one of the top-rated lighters on the market. A downside of the ubiquitous, popular cigarette lighters, however, is their sometimes-unreliable sparking mechanism under inclement weather conditions. In the world of matches and lighters, the UCO Stormproof butane "stormproof" lighter is highly rated, and not just water-resistant, but waterproof.

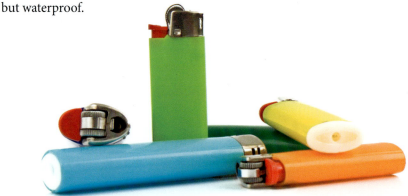

Signaling Devices

Depending on the nature of your travels, you may wish to equip yourself or party with some additional, professional emergency signaling devices. I've purchased a Sportsmen's Signal Kit, and a ACR Firefly Rescue Lite because I spend time in some of the most remote parts of Canada where extra precautions are warranted. The first kit is no longer manufactured, but its components or facsimiles can still be purchased.

Whistles

There are several types of commercial whistles (e.g., police, dog, train, referee and factory) and other natural whistles (e.g., pucker, finger, hand, teeth and roof) all of which can be used to sound an alarm, stay in touch with trail companions or call for help. These varieties of whistles have different pitches. They are used to attract attention and are great survival tools (more on p. 215).

Sportsmen's Signal Kit

The Sportsmen's Signal Kit was manufactured by Survival Systems, Inc. and contains two Skyblazers red aerial flare/launchers that fire a magnesium meteor flare to high altitudes. It also contains a SMOKE cannister that can be activated by removing the cap and then thrown in the water or used on land to signal your whereabouts. In addition, the kit contains a cannister which holds water resistant matches, a striker, tinder, fire starter and an instruction sheet. Skyblazers aerial flares can be ordered online (see Appendix).

ACR Firefly Rescue Lite

Several years ago, I purchased this pocket-sized, handheld, military grade strobe light, which provides many square miles of nighttime visibility as a signaling device. It penetrates rain and fog where conventional flashlights fail. The unit is capable of operating for nine continuous hours, much longer if used intermittently. It is constructed of rugged, shock-resistant material to withstand adverse field conditions. There is a new ACR Firefly PRO Solas emergency strobe light model (see Appendix) that operates for up to 56 hours of use and features AA lithium batteries.

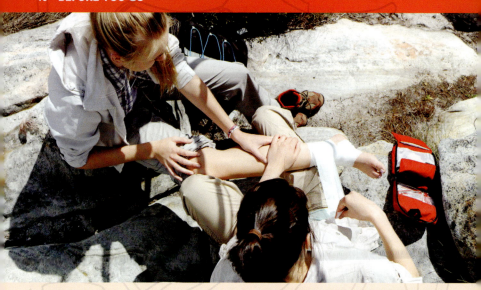

First Aid Kit

Every outdoorsperson should have a first aid kit: a pocket-size kit for personal use in the field and another commercial/industrial kit for camp use or to keep in your vehicle if you're travelling in remote areas. The most important contents of a pocket-size first aid kit can help to stop bleeding from a wound and prevent infections arising from cuts and bruises. First aid kits can be purchased in a variety of sizes, or they can be custom made if you want to make your own kit.

You never know when you are going to need first aid when you're in the bush. On a fly-in fishing trip to the remote Upper Toobally Lake, Yukon, I had the misfortune of being impaled with a barbless hook through the index finger on my left hand—believe me when I say, that hurts! I always carry a Leatherman multi-tool when fishing, which I used to remove the hook that had gone right through my finger and out the other side (it was a large-sized streamer hook). Next, I treated the wound with some antiseptic, bandaged it and went on fishing! While the wound was painful for a while, the pain didn't last very long. I had some pain killers, but I didn't feel a need to use them. However, without the first aid kit on hand, things could have been a lot worse.

For camp (or vehicle) purposes, I recommend a commercial kit that contains contents for injuries that are more serious than what you are likely to experience during a day trip where a pocket-size kit should be adequate. I suggest purchasing a quality commercial first aid kit from the Safety Supply Company, which has branches across Canada for all-purpose camp/workplace needs, or another reputable company. Below is a list of the typical contents of both types of kits.

Pocket-size First Aid Kit Components (for day use)

- Bandages and knuckle dressings in assorted sizes
- Adhesive sterile wound dressing
- Sting relief
- Benzalkonium chloride serviette, antiseptic compound towelettes
- APAP (non-aspirin pain relie)

Commercial First Aid Kit Components (for camp, workplace or vehicle)

- First aid kit handbook
- Instruments (medical)
- Eye dressing packet
- Polysporin
- Pressure dressing
- Ammonia inhalants
- Metal splint
- Sting-Stop swabs
- Burn compound
- Merthiolate swabs
- Triangular bandage
- Compress bandage
- Adhesive bandage
- Gauze bandages
- Waterproof adhesive tape
- Surgical tape

Sunscreen

Don't leave home without sunscreen. Apply it before you head outdoors and be sure to reapply throughout the day, especially if you are perspiring.

Bug Spray

Insect spray is essential in Canada's boreal forest and especially in Yukon, Northwest Territories and Nunavut. Mosquitos are probably the worst insects, followed by blackflies and deer flies. While Yukon tends to be drier than either the Northwest Territories or Nunavut it too has lots of mosquitoes in wetted areas.

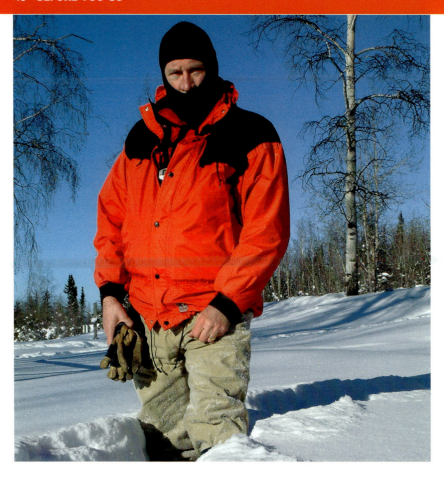

Clothing and Footwear

The saga of John Hornby's travels stands testament to the importance of appropriate outdoor and cold weather clothing and footwear. Apparel must be warm, comfortable, as lightweight as possible, wind and waterproof and preferably layered so it can be put on and taken off as conditions change.

Nowadays, it is generally standard practice to dress in layers. If the weather is likely going to be cool or cold, start with a base layer of undergarments, leggings and t-shirt, made out of polyester. The top and bottom will serve to keep you warm

Dress in layers. The weather can change quickly, so it is important that you choose the proper clothing and footwear so you can be prepared.

but will wick away sweat which otherwise chills the body. Next, wear some comfortable cargo pants; there are many styles available that stretch and are waterproof. Wear a long-sleeved shirt, preferably of polyester material that stretches and keeps heat in your torso. These outer garments are surprisingly warm. A lightweight, water-repellant wind breaker jacket is usually adequate for day trips in the Canadian summer, supplemented by a long or short sleeve fleece vest for days when it's cool outside.

Legend has it that Inuit understood the importance of dressing in layers with windproof outer garments to stay warm in sub-zero temperatures. Inuit traditionally wore an anorak over top of inner layers for centuries to combat cold weather. Inuit also realized the danger of working up a sweat, which could exacerbate the danger of hypothermia. Hypothermia occurs when a person's body loses heat faster than it can generate it, causing a dangerously low body temperature that can result in death.

I have spent a lifetime researching and testing outdoor apparel and compact, lightweight gear to maximize my mobility—in comfort—while in Canada's great outdoors. The key to a successful trip is to stay dry and warm. However, when you are not overloaded with bulky and heavy clothing, your outdoor adventures will be even more rewarding.

Synthetics have revolutionized outdoor apparel starting with boots that are not only very light but also waterproof, warm and durable, with ankle support and good traction. Next come socks that provide warmth and cushioned soles for added comfort. New polyester and wool base layers (i.e., underwear) are not only warm, but practically weightless; then there are synthetic outdoor pants that are waterproof, windproof and that shed burrs.

Legend has it that Inuit understood the importance of dressing in layers with windproof outer garments to stay warm in sub-zero temperatures.

The key to a successful and enjoyable trip is to stay dry and warm.

There's no going back for something you've forgotten when you are hundreds of kilometres away from your home.

Three key synthetic products have revolutionized the outdoor apparel market: Gore-Tex®, Polar fleece and Thinsulate®.

Gore-Tex® is a waterproof/breathable fabric characterized by a porous form of polytetrafluoroethylene (the chemical constituent of Teflon) with a micro-structure characterized by nodes interconnected by fibrils: a "waterproof laminate." Windproof and waterproof outdoor jackets made of Gore-Tex® are the norm in today's outdoor apparel marketplace.

From microfleece to heavyweight, **Polar fleece**, usually referred to simply as "fleece," is a soft napped insulating synthetic fabric made from polyethylene terephthalate (PET) or other synthetic fibers. It is a soft, lightweight, warm and comfortable fabric. It is hydrophobic, holding less than 1% of its weight in water, retains much of its insulating powers even when wet and it is highly breathable.

Thinsulate™ is a microfabric made from synthetic fibers, woven together in various thicknesses, that helps keep you warm in sub-zero temperatures. The Thinsulate™ brand is a trademark of the 3M Corporation. The word is a portmanteau of *thin* and *insulate*. Apparel made of this fabric is noted for being both very light and warm. I'm sold on Thinsulate™ clothing because it is warm and lightweight, ideal for Canada's outdoors.

Now, it appears as though a new generation of insulated down jackets that feature Omni-Heat® Thermal Reflective material is going to take outdoor apparel to yet another level with manufacturers claims of garments being at least 20 percent warmer because of this new technology. The thermal reflective technology helps regulate your temperature by reflecting and retaining the warmth your body generates while dissipating moisture and excess heat to keep you comfortable. Field tests indicate that Omni-Heat® Thermal Reflective insulated hunting jackets and bibs are incredibly warm, quiet and breathable, which is more good news for outdoorspeople.

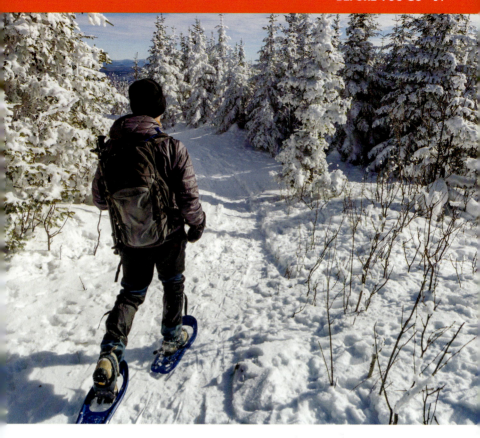

When it's –15°C or colder with a wind blowing, you must be prepared for bone-chilling events. Your life depends on it. This is the temperature threshold I have set for myself based on personal experience in the outdoors, though others might have more tolerance than me. I have developed a checklist that I use to gear up for such conditions because it is vitally important to be prepared for the worst weather, especially if you're travelling some distance from home. Below zero temperatures with high wind chills can stretch for a week or more. There's no going back for something you've forgotten when you are hundreds of kilometres away from your home. It is also very important to have lightweight apparel—not heavy, bulky clothing—to be mobile and avoid overexerting yourself.

When it's –15°C or colder with a wind blowing, you must be prepared for bone-chilling events. Your life depends on it.

Layering

People of different ages have different tolerances to weather. Some might be better adapted to cold weather, while others are not. It is important that you consider your personal tolerance when reviewing the following checklist, which is my list of necessary gear when temperatures plummet.

- I wear a polyester base layer (top and bottom) that wicks sweat away when temperatures are near 0°C.
- I switch to a Marino wool undergarment base layer at −10°C temperatures or lower.
- I wear lightweight winter boots that feature Thinsulate™ lining rated for −32°C, have good ankle support and traction, among other key features.
- I wear microfleece pants at sub-zero temperatures, but if there is a significant wind chill I'll switch to GORE-TEX® lined pants, the ultimate for cold weather when matched with Marino wool undergarments.
- I wear Marino wool winter socks (not cotton) because they have cushioning and wicking fibers.
- If snow is more than ankle deep, I'll put on gaiters to keep the snow out of my boots which will otherwise chill your feet when it melts.
- There are many thermal sweatshirts on the market that are ideal for sub-zero temperature.
- Depending on how cold it is, I'll wear either a sleeveless and/or long-sleeved fleece liner vest, light and warm. (A waterproof down vest is another option.)
- I wear a hooded Thinsulate™ parka with storm cuffs that is both warm and made of fabric that is lightweight. A fur-lined hood offers the ultimate protection.
- I wear Thinsulate™ mittens and carry wool gloves with and without fingers that I can switch to if I need to use my fingers when it is very cold.
- To keep my head warm, I wear either a microfibre tuque or a Thinsulate™ hat depending on just how cold it is.
- I always pack a woollen balaclava for extremely cold weather which can be a life saver to prevent frostbite on my ears, nose and face if there is any amount of wind.

Outdoorspeople are especially susceptible to both frostbite and hypothermia because of frigid weather that is common during Canadian winters. It is fairly routine to have to travel long distances with a backpack, which can cause a person to sweat. Then, as a person's body cools off, their body temperature drops, and their fingers and toes get cold. This can lead to both frostbite and hypothermia. You must be properly dressed, or you should not even be in the outdoors under such conditions. The dangers of snow and cold temperatures should never be taken for granted. Once hypothermia starts, the patient must be taken care of quickly or they will die of exposure (see Hypothermia on page 146).

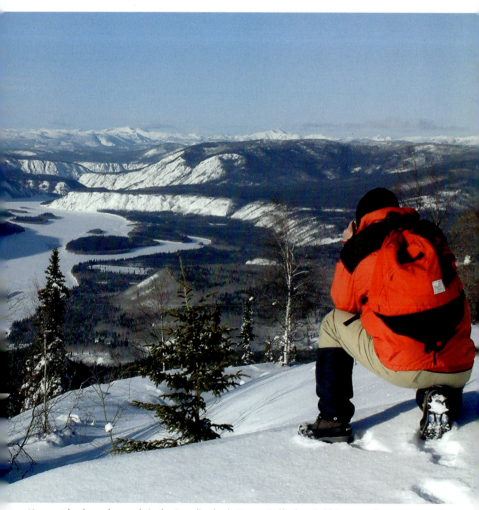

You must be dressed properly in the Canadian bush. Duane Radford on Gold Dome Lookout, Dawson City, Yukon, overlooking the Yukon River.

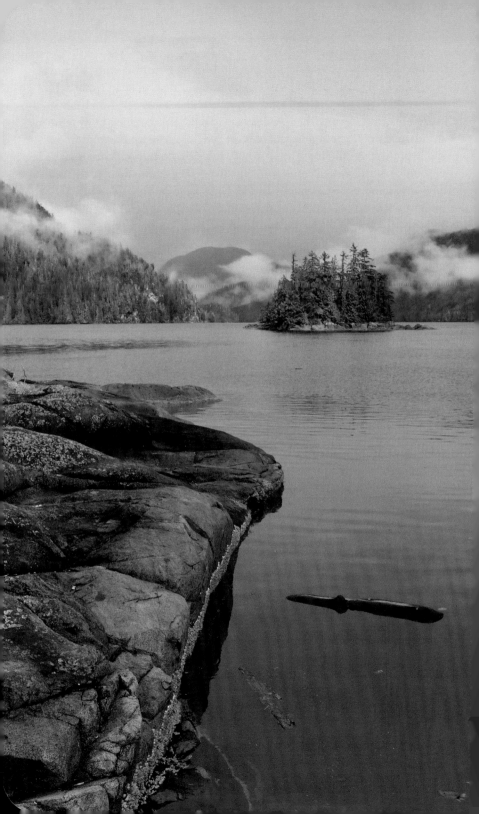

Raingear

Don't leave home for a long hike without raingear. In the mountains of Alberta and British Columbia, it's typically bright and sunny in the morning, but as the day warms up, clouds will form and can develop into thunderstorms. There's nothing worse than getting drenched in the outdoors.

Hats

You should always wear a hat in the outdoors to minimize the danger of heat stroke and ward off skin cancer. While a baseball cap is okay, a hat with a wide brim is better to shade your eyes.

Sunglasses

It is important to bring sunglasses to protect your eyes. While most sunglasses provide 100 percent UV protection, I highly recommend using polarized sunglasses for both protection and better visibility.

Leather Gloves

Leather gloves are must-have items for outdoorspeople, especially those who are planning to camp or spend extended time in the outdoors. They are useful for cutting and stacking wood for campfires and for constructing backcountry shelters. They will shield your hands from rough wood, or you may otherwise get splinters that can become infected. Likewise, leather gloves ward against thorns that might cause infections in your fingers and hands. They will also help provide a better grip when using axes and when handling rough and/or large objects such as logs and boulders that may need to be moved about in a campsite. They also come in handy when setting up a tent and pounding in tent pegs.

Nowadays, you don't necessarily need "leather" gloves, because most forms of work gloves will do the same job and are quite sturdy. There are lots of durable, inexpensive work gloves on the market that are available in Canadian big box stores such as Canadian Tire and Mark's Work Warehouse.

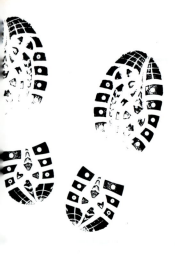

Footwear

I rate quality, leather boots with **Vibram** soles as the best all-around footwear for travel in the spring, summer and autumn. The vulcanized sole is designed to provide excellent traction on the widest ranges of surfaces. When treated, leather is waterproof and provides excellent ankle support for walking on slopes and uneven surfaces. Hiking boots made of synthetic fibers are light and comfortable, but don't meet the standards of leather boots; further, they're not always waterproof. It's important to tighten your laces to provide solid ankle support and minimize blisters. Finish with a double knot so laces don't come loose and check laces periodically to make sure they're tight.

Almost all leather boots require a break-in period so your feet can get accustomed to the new, stiff leather. If you don't break-in new boots before a hike, you will develop blisters. It is always a good idea to go on a series of short hikes to break in new boots before going on long hikes. Boots that are made of synthetic material do not require a similar, lengthy break-in period.

I prefer hiking socks made from piled synthetic fibers or Merino wool which are breathable, light, soft, warm and comfortable. These features are important for day long hikes. Socks must be the right size or you will get a blister. On long hikes, I take a spare pair and change them for the hike back to the trailhead. Try to pace yourself on longer hikes; don't rush, because that's when accidents happen.

It is always a good idea to go on a series of short hikes to break in new boots before going on long hikes.

Waterproofing Your Gear

I'd highly recommend that any outside apparel be made of waterproof material, which shouldn't be a challenge to locate what with all of the modern outdoor garments now available. If your clothing is not made of waterproof material, there are many commercial waterproof spray products on today's market. Products like "Scotch Guard Outdoor Water Shield" have been available for many years and there are dozens of similar spray products to treat fabrics that are not waterproof. Footwear, however, is another matter as most footwear is not completely waterproofed at time of purchase.

I've opted for leather hiking boots with Vibram soles for 50+ years and have never regretted this choice, because on the occasions I've worn hiking boots made of synthetic material I've found they are not fully waterproof. Leather is sturdy and provides ideal ankle support, better than synthetic boots. Granted, synthetic boots are light, comfortable, warm and sturdy, but water can get through the fibers. When this happens, they will stay wet inside all day and must be dried out 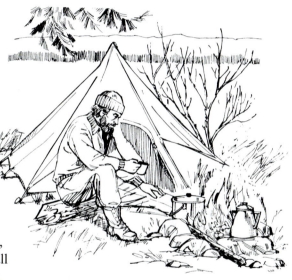 because they lose their insulating properties. However, I will use gaiters if necessary when conditions warrant and when wearing leather boots is unnecessary because waterproofing isn't an issue, especially in deep snow, and boots made of synthetic material are suitable.

New leather boots should be treated with commercial waterproofing wax for leather products as required. In my case, one treatment is good for extended periods afield. However, after applying the waterproofing compound to my leather boots, I also spray them with an aerosol waterproofing spray to provide added protection against water and stains. Boots should be cleaned with soapy water and must be dry before applying either waterproofing wax or spray for best results.

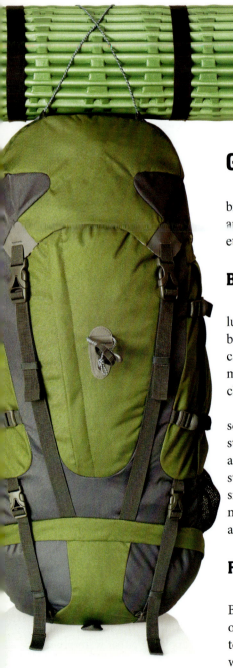

Gear

Intro about how the gear you choose to bring will depend on the type of trip you are taking (i.e., length, location, purpose, etc.).

Backpacks

A day pack is necessary to store your lunch, high energy snacks and water. The brand you select should be chosen with care, depending on your needs. There are many different styles on the market to choose from.

Don't leave home without packing sunscreen—remember to apply it before you start your hike—and a pocket flashlight and waterproof matches in case you get stranded. I also take a space blanket and signal flares for emergencies; while I've never used them, they do provide insurance if necessary.

Flashlights and Headlamps

Outdoor Canada Hunting Editor, Ken Bailey, says a source of light (i.e., flashlight or headlamp) has proven to be comforting to people who are lost overnight or otherwise spending time in the dark. Make sure it's waterproof and lightweight, and don't forget some extra batteries.

Flashlights

There are many compact flashlights on the market that are easy to carry and have proven indispensable to me while hiking out of remote areas in the dark.

Headlamps

A quality headlamp is invaluable, freeing up your hands while trekking on known trails and completing any number of other chores, including signaling in emergency situations.

Headlamps are especially useful in cases where it is necessary to walk on game trails at night, which is not uncommon for hunters in particular. They will free up your hands to use trekking poles if the terrain is challenging instead of holding a flashlight in one of your hands. Hunters also find them indispensable for field dressing downed big game animals in the dark and as signaling devices to locate other members in a hunting party.

It is important to remove batteries from headlamps when not in use so as to prevent corrosion. They should be checked for battery strength before heading afield, and at least one set of spare batteries should be packed for emergencies. There are, however, rechargeable battery-operated headlamps and a wide variety of headlamps available in today's market. They have been labelled as being "bright, versatile and indispensable" for good reason and should be in every outdoorsperson's pack.

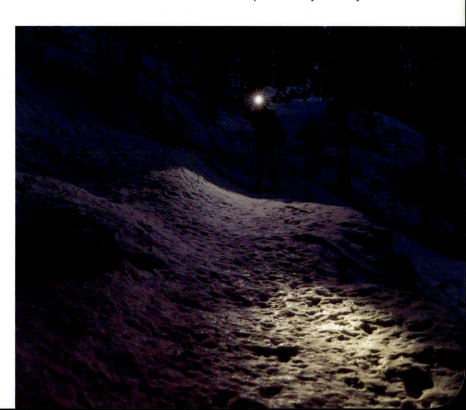

Trekking Poles

When hiking, trekking poles are recommended for all adults, seniors in particular. They're like extra appendages and will provide balance on slopes and rough ground. Take at least one extendable trekking pole, two if you're in the mountains.

Snowshoes

There is a long history of snowshoeing in Canada. Many parts of Canada's boreal forest get heavy snowfall (4-5+ feet) during the winter. In Newfoundland, 8+ feet may fall in parts of the northern peninsula. The mountainous areas in western Canada can get even more snowfall (up to 20+ feet). It is virtually impossible to walk on top of this much snow, and usually the only way to get around is by wearing snowshoes. Even with snowshoes, however, travel is difficult—especially for a person who has to break a new trail. Indigenous Peoples, early explorers and fur trappers used snowshoes to travel during the winter months. Even dog sled teams get bogged down by heavy snow and may not be able to travel unless a trail is broken for them by a person on snowshoes.

Modern snowshoes are much lighter than the old hardwood varieties, often with aluminum frames, and are available in a number of sizes and shapes. Bindings and buckles have evolved to include ratchets or quick clips. Metal crampons on the bottom of modern snowshoes help with walking up hills and crossing icy sections.

Mountain Equipment Cooperative has an online chart that provides general recommendations for sizing snowshoes. Generally speaking, the most popular size of snowshoe is between 25 and 27 inches long and between 9 and 10 inches wide. These are recommended for people who weigh up to approximately 195 pounds. Snowshoes specifically made for women are 22 to 25 inches long and between 7 and 8 inches wide.

There are several popular, basic types of snowshoes in Canada: Huron/Algonquin, Bearpaw and Cree/Ojibwe with different sizes recommended for adult and youth as outlined by the Lure of the North online (see Appendix).

Huron/Algonquin Snowshoes

Huron/Algonquin snowshoes have a classic "teardrop" shape with a rounded, up-turned toe and a long tail. They are both wide and long and are the Lure of The North favourite "travelling" snowshoe. That is, they do well in open country and on lakes, rivers, marshes and fields. The tail serves two functions: it stabilizes the shoe to keep it from twisting on your foot, and it acts as a counterweight so that the toe naturally crests deep snow.

Bearpaw (left) and Huron (right) snowshoes

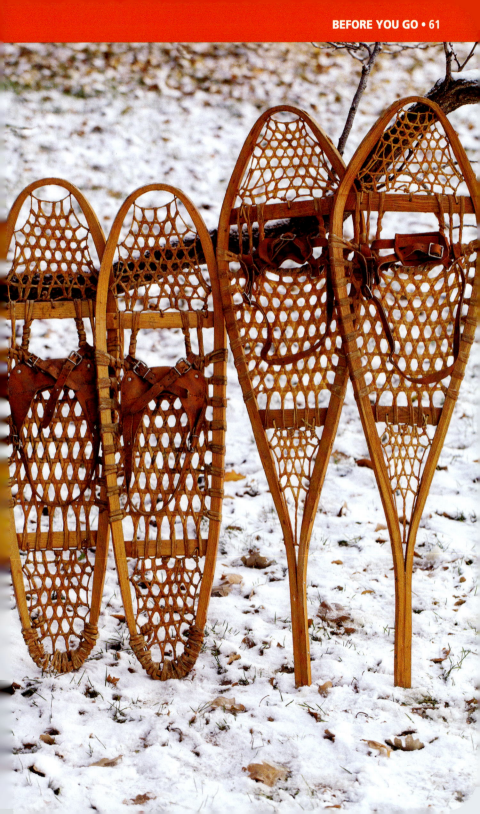

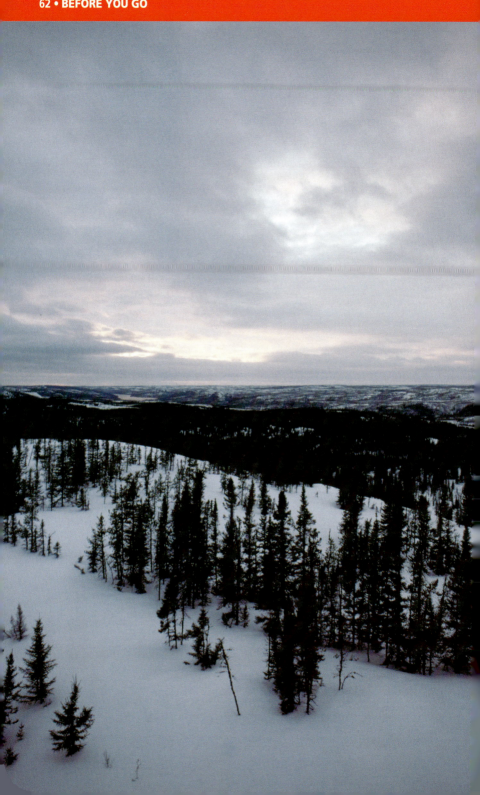

Bearpaw Snowshoes

Bearpaw snowshoes are short and wide, with a round toe and no tail. These are the favourite Lure of the North "bush" or "camp" shoes. They do exceptionally well in forested country and are great around camp or when trapping, hunting or gathering wood. Without a tail, these shoes are much more evenly balanced than Huron shoes. This also means that the toes do not crest deep snow as well as Huron shoes, but it is much easier to lift the heel of the shoe to turn or back up.

Cree/Ojibwe Snowshoes

Cree/Ojibwe snowshoes are easily recognized as a snowshoe native to much of northern Ontario. These shoes are long and narrow, with both a tail and a pointed, up-turned toe. These shoes can be great for fast travel in open country; however, Lure of the North is of the opinion that commercially available frames in this style are all too narrow. They maintain that very narrow frames lack lateral stability (i.e., they tend to dive sideways into the snow) and do not pack a great "float" or trail for a toboggan to follow in. They advise that while travelling along the James Bay coast of Northern Quebec they saw Indigenous-made Cree-style snowshoes, which were wider than commercial frames, that did not seem to suffer this disadvantage.

James Bay, Northern Quebec

My uncle Carl Sapeta gave me a pair of Ojibwe snowshoes when I was growing up in southwestern Alberta in the Rocky Mountains. Carl was an outdoorsman who hunted and prospected in Alberta and the Northwest Territories. He also had a registered trapline on Vicary Creek in the Crowsnest Forest Reserve north of his home in Coleman, where he snowshoed to get around on his trapline. The frames of the Ojibwe snowshoes were made of hardwood with leather bindings. Deep snow was common when I was a kid, and I used these snowshoes to get around in the outdoors. I developed a respect for the Indigenous Peoples who invented them as a means of winter travel. The snowshoes imitated nature's way of getting around in deep snow. For example, snowshoe hares and Canada lynx both have large, padded feet so they can walk on top of deep snow. Ruffed grouse have tufts of feathers on their feet for the same purpose—to increase the surface area of their feet and better distribute their weight.

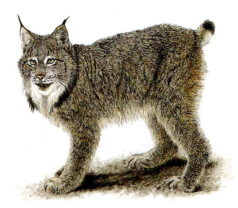

Snowshoeing can be very challenging and exhausting. Long stints have been known to cause "mal de raquette," which can be seriously disabling, causing lameness in worst case scenarios. While the idea behind snowshoes is to distribute a person's weight over a larger area, even a snowshoe will settle into snow with each step necessitating energy to lift it and step forward. This repetitive movement can be very tiring and even people in good physical conditions can find it exhausting. One of the hidden dangers is breaking out into a sweat which dampens clothing that can be difficult to dry out. Wet clothing will not hold heat and can lead to hypothermia.

Snowshoeing was traditionally done over river courses and trails where bush wasn't an obstacle and requires a lot of skill to get around off trail. Snowshoeing remains popular to this day with an array of versatile products available, and it has shown a renaissance in recent years with a variety of new, quality snowshoes coming into the market.

Flares

Originally, I purchased a compact ERMA SG67E hand-held flare launcher that is similar to the "Tru Friend Pen Launcher" advertised in Mountain Equipment Co-op. It is practically indestructible. This pen-sized launcher can fire flares or noise-making bear bangers. I also have a spare Stare Blazer launcher that I use exclusively to hold bear bangers. Hand-held flare launchers and flares can be found in many Canadian sporting goods stores besides outlets such as Mountain Equipment Co-op.

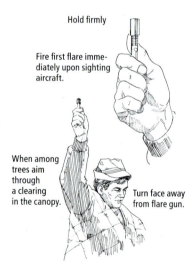

Hold firmly

Fire first flare immediately upon sighting aircraft.

When among trees aim through a clearing in the canopy.

Turn face away from flare gun.

Most flare launchers are compact, pencil shaped devices that fit in your pocket. The small flares come in different colors such as red to signal danger or green to signal that you're okay. When hiking or fishing I routinely carry a flare launcher loaded with a bear banger and some spare bangers as back up. Bear banger flares explode at a range of approximately 50 feet. With a little practice they are surprising accurate. Flare guns come with firing instructions.

Flares are dangerous and should only be used by adults. Because they are flammable, they should be used with caution because they could start a forest or grass fire.

Special Tools (Leatherman) and Knives

In addition to my personalized survival kit, I always pack a Leatherman Pocket Survival Tool kit in a sheath (that can fit on my belt), along with at least one extra pocketknife. (Note: a small knife is in the *Survival Kit* on page 40).

I am an angler and hunter, and I often need a multi-purpose tool kit to make equipment repairs when I'm in the outdoors. I have found that the Leatherman Pocket Survival Tool is one of the better kits on the market for this purpose, and it can also be used in a pinch to make repairs on outboard motors and around camp. During a fishing trip to the Cree River Lodge in northern Saskatchewan, my guide hit a hard object in the Cree River that broke off part of the propeller blade. Amazingly, my son, Myles, found the missing part in the muskeg stained river which was remarkable considering that the Cree River such a large river. Without the Leatherman special tool kit, we would never have been able to repair the

It is essential that you have some kind of survival tool kit to make emergency repairs and to deal with other contingencies.

propeller blade and get back to camp, which was dozens of miles away with no help nearby. It is essential that you have some kind of survival tool kit to make emergency repairs and to deal with other contingencies.

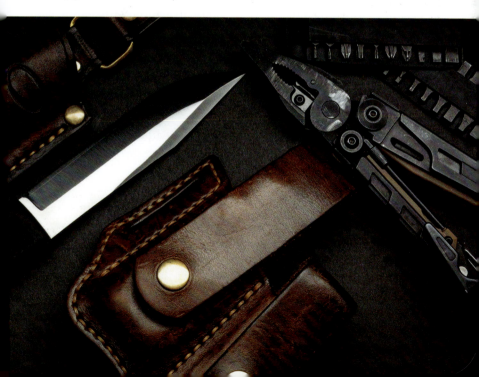

My Leatherman kit features needle nose pliers and wire cutters. The pliers and wire cutters are ideal for setting wire snares (more details in *Porcupines, Fool Hens, Animal Snares and Traps* on page 131). You can also use the pliers to dislodge a fishing hook that is impaled in a person's body—believe me that this is not uncommon. The Leatherman has a knife, wood/metal file, Phillips screwdriver and a tool adapter with custom hex and other screwdriver bits. There are other similar brands on the market, so I suggest you shop around to find one that best serves your particular needs.

A multitude of hunting knives are available for today's outdoorsperson to suit a variety of purposes, but they don't always fall into a survival category.

Filleting knives are another story. As a hunter, I've long been sold on the Browning folding 3-bladed knife, which features a skinning blade, a hide-cutter blade and a bone cutting saw. Other outdoorspeople prefer a knife that only has a skinning blade. Even though I use a Browning knife to field dress a big game animal, I fall back on Victorinox professional quality boning and skinning knives to get their hide off and debone an animal.

However, for all-around camp purposes, there is no substitute for a quality pocketknife, and there are many good brands on the market. Two of my favourite brands of pocketknives, which have many different styles, are the Old Timer and Victorinox Swiss Army because of their high quality and versatility. Unfortunately, the Old Timer brand is no longer in production, so if you have one, it is considered a genuine classic to be treasured. The Swiss Army knives have an array of useful features that come in handy and have been on the market for many years.

Pick a pocketknife that's functional; it doesn't have to have a multitude of gadgets, just ones that are useful. A small honing steel to realign blade edges and a knife sharpener to bring back the edge on blades are necessary. Before leaving home, ensure that the blades of your pocket knife are sharpened.

> **A multitude of hunting knives are available for today's outdoorsperson to suit a variety of purposes, but they don't always fall into a survival category.**

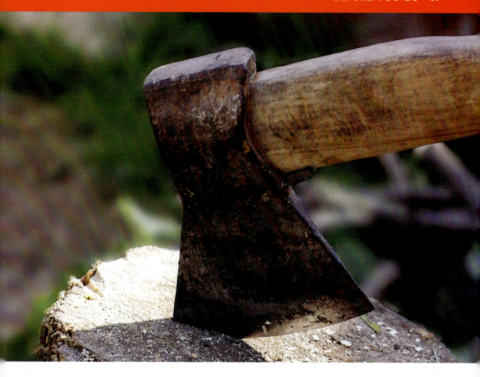

Axes, Hatchets and Saws

Axes

There are many brands of axes on today's market that will be adequate for outdoor survival, so it is important to know what you are using your axe for. An axe comes in handy for cutting branches off trees to clear an area for camping, chopping firewood, getting rid of troublesome roots where you intend to pitch a tent and pounding in tent pegs.

Cutting axes have a shallow wedge angle, whereas splitting axes have a deeper angle. Most axes are double beveled (i.e., symmetrical about the axis of the blade). These are among the most popular axes for outdoor use.

Axes are used for both cutting and splitting wood (cutting is against the wood grain, while splitting is along the wood grain). A cutting/chopping axe is ideal for most outdoor purposes

Cutting or chopping axes are ideal for outdoor use.

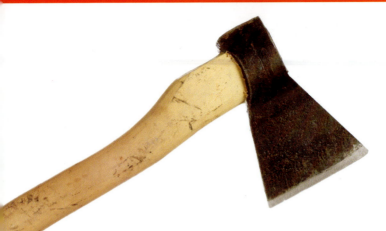

because they are generally lighter and smaller than a splitting axe. Pick an axe with a handle length that you're comfortable with, keeping in mind that an axe with a longer handle is generally safer to use.

The blade shape in axe heads come in two basic varieties: curved and flat blades. The sharper the curve of the blade, the more the blade will penetrate the wood. An axe blade with some curve will have better versatility than a flat edge. I suggest a single-bit axe head, not a double-bit, for survival purposes for reasons of safety and practicality.

Axe Care

You will need a steel file to sharpen the axe and a leather sheath (or blade cover) to protect the axe head and ensure it does not damage your gear. A dull axe can be dangerous because it can bounce off the surface, potentially causing injury. Ensure the blade is sharp and protect wooden axe handles with a coating of boiled linseed oil to prevent splintering. Store axes with wooden handles securely when not in camp; porcupines have been known to chew up axe handles in search of salt.

Hatchets

While you will need two hands to wield an axe properly, hatchets are meant to be used with one hand. Generally, hatchets aren't an ideal survival tool because they're not constructed to chop down large trees or split firewood; they're simply too small for this job. I have, however, used a hatchet for backpacking on many occasions because they're compact, lightweight and perfectly adequate for all-purpose camp duties, so long as the weather isn't extreme.

Saws and Bow (Swede) Saws

A bow saw (or Swede saw) is a metal-framed crosscut saw in the shape of a bow with a coarse, wide blade that should be in every outdoor camp. These practical saws are indispensable for all-purpose camp duties, every bit or even more important and versatile than axes and hatchets. You can easily cut through logs and trees up to six inches in diameter with a bow saw in a matter of just minutes. They come in different sizes and are compact and easy to carry and store. They can be used to build emergency shelters and cut firewood with ease. These versatile saws come with 21-, 24- and 30-inch blades, depending on their intended purpose. There are several different brands of bow saws on the market to choose from. I've used bow saws my whole life and wouldn't venture into the outdoors on a camping trip without one.

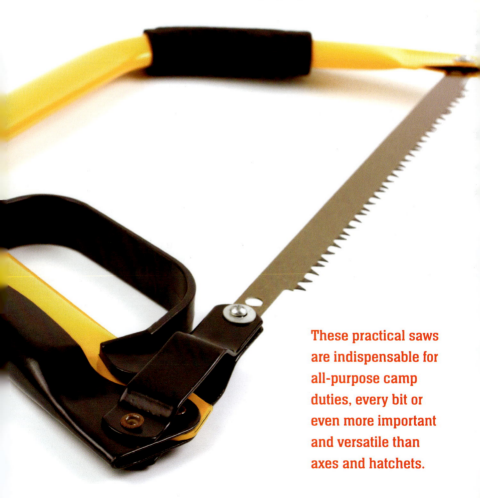

These practical saws are indispensable for all-purpose camp duties, every bit or even more important and versatile than axes and hatchets.

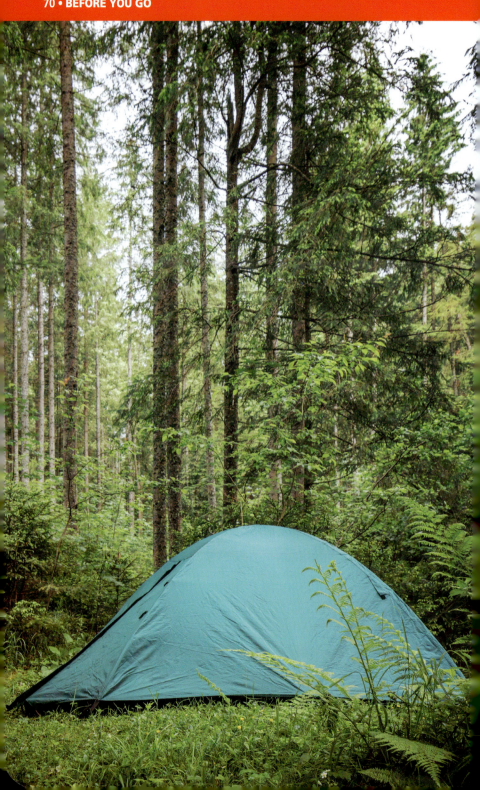

Tents

Tents are synonymous with camping in Canada and often key to survival in the wild. A tent keeps you and your gear dry, warm and sheltered from the elements. It also provides protection from insects, as most tents have an awning and built-in mosquito bar.

Wall Tents

In Canada, wall tents have long been popular with early explorers, geologists, hunters and trail riders, primarily because they're quite comfortable and roomy. They've been made of canvas since time immemorial—although cotton can also be substituted for canvas—and can be treated with a waterproofing compound to repel rain and snow.

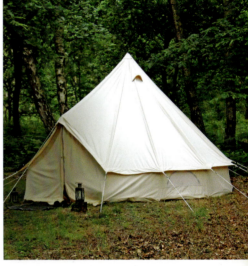

Old style wall tents required a ridge pole to keep the roof up, while the sides were anchored to the ground by canvas loops along the base of the walls with spikes driven into the ground. These tents did not have a canvas floor, and the ridge pole was tied to a couple of trees.

New models of wall tents have a brace for the ridge pole. Nylon is used in new wall tents that are framed with aluminum poles, and new models can be equipped with a fly. Typically, the tents will be heated with a small, portable wood stove. This is called an "airtight" stove that can quickly warm a large tent and can also be used for cooking. It should be noted that a tent will not hold heat, and a stove must be fed a supply of wood to keep it warm.

A downside of canvas wall tents is that they are bulky and heavy. They can be freighted in boats and canoes or by planes or horses. The old-fashioned wall tents are ideal for waiting out a storm

A catalytic heater is a flameless heater that uses a chemical reaction instead of a flame to produce heat, although they do use propane to fuel the reaction. There is no flame or fire, so they are safe to use in a camping tent, and they do not produce any dangerous carbon monoxide. Heaters that use methanol for fuel, however, should only be used in well ventilated situations.

in relative comfort but don't always stand up well in strong, persistent windstorms.

Nowadays, most tents are made of nylon that is light, waterproof, easy to repair if torn and comes equipped with a built-in fly to keep out rain. As well as nylon, Egyptian cotton has long been a popular material for tents because it has some water-repellent properties when wet.

Typically, it's not safe to use a woodstove in a nylon tent, and if necessary, they should be heated with a catalytic heater. Otherwise, there's a risk of carbon monoxide poisoning. When heating a tent with a stove, it is better to have a canvas tent, which is less flammable than nylon.

Nylon tents are light and easy to pack, and most are easy to set up and don't require any special gear. Keep in mind, unless well anchored, they can blow away in a wind. As well, most backpacking tents, while easy to pack and carry, are small and somewhat cramped.

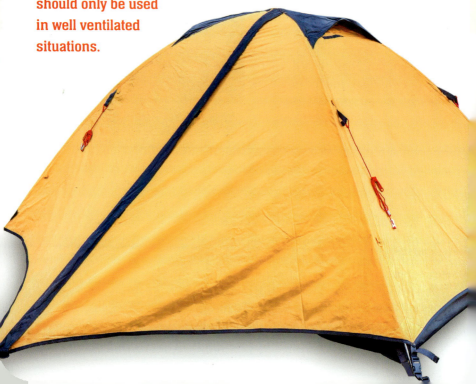

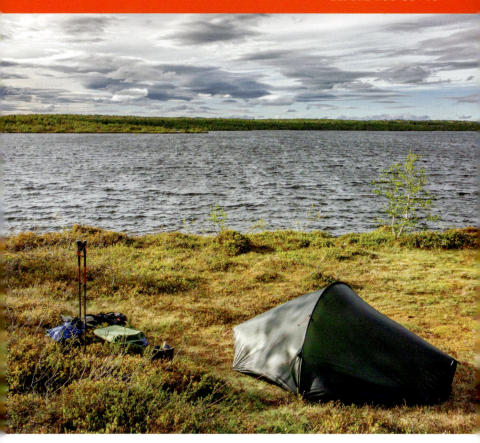

Mountaineer's Tent

A mountaineer's tent is made of nylon and comes in handy for a person who only requires a place to sleep with protection from the elements. They're very small and lightweight with a floor sewn into the walls to keep out night drafts and insects. These tents are compact with only enough room for a sleeping bag and a very small amount of gear, making them a good option for shorter trips.

Tarps

A tarp is also a useful item to have in camp to cover gear and wood, so it stays dry, or to use as a windbreak, etc. There are also different types of makeshift "tents" you can fashion out of a tarp including the *forester's tent* and the *lean-to tent* (see Shelter building on page 104).

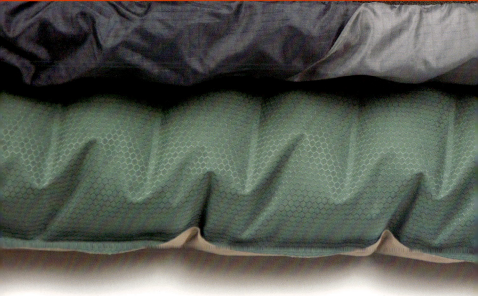

Sleeping Bags and Mattresses

Sleeping Bags

Nowadays, the two most popular insulations in sleeping bags are down and synthetic, having long ago replaced cotton batting. I have used bags with both kinds of insulation, and both have good billings.

Sleeping bags typically come in mummy and old-school standard (regular) shapes, although barrel shaped bags are also marketed. Some standard shaped bags can be used alone and/or zippered together. Most salespeople claim that a mummy bag is warmer than a regular bag; however, I think this a matter of personal preference. An issue I have with the mummy bag is that my legs are confined, which is true for most tall people, so I don't have as good a sleep compared with a barrel shaped bag.

The size and weight of these two kinds of bags are key features that should be considered before purchasing a sleeping bag, as well as the temperature ratings, which are subjective.

Down

Down bags are lightweight, compact, warm and durable, though they won't be as comfortable in humid or wet environments. Compaction of down over time—especially if not stored properly—and loss of insulating values if the down gets wet are issues. I've had down bags get wet when packhorses have stumbled and fell into the water when fording mountain streams, submerging the bags in cold water. It takes a long time for a wet down bag to dry out.

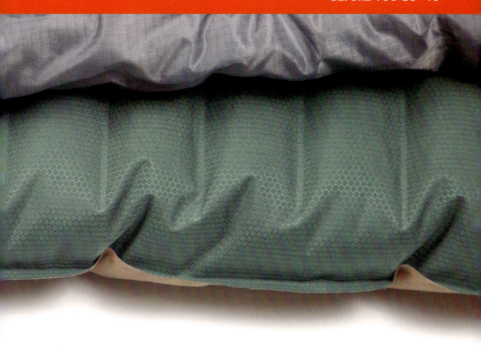

Synthetic

Reviews indicate that synthetic sleeping bags tend to be more affordable, heavier and bulkier. They are often better than their down counterparts when it comes to keeping you warm in a humid climate such as the Coastal Mountain Range of British Columbia, which experiences heavy precipitation. Synthetic bags are also the only option for those who are allergic to down feathers. However, synthetic bags often weigh a bit more than down bags and are a bit bulkier, which is an issue for backpackers.

DOWN	SYNTHETIC
Lightweight	Warm
Compact	More affordable
Compresses better than synthetic material	Heavier and bulkier than down
Not good for damp climates and takes a long time to dry	Good for damp climates and dry more quickly than down

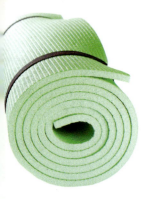

Mattresses

Sleeping pads or air mattress do add insulation and comfort when camping in the Canadian outdoors where freezing temperatures are not uncommon, especially in the mountains of Western Canada—even during the summer months. Expect to see ice on top of the water bucket in the morning.

It is true that your bag will provide some insulation under your body when compressed, but it won't stay as warm when you're sleeping on a pad or mattress. My advice is to purchase the best sleeping bag that you can afford, along with a ground mattress that compliments the type of use you have in mind (i.e. backpacking, camping, etc.). Keep in mind that just about all unheated tents have condensation issues overnight, and dampness can impact the insulating properties of your sleeping bag (down bags in particular).

You will not have a comfortable sleep unless you have a warm sleeping bag, but even the best bags need a mattress if you are sleeping on the cold, hard ground.

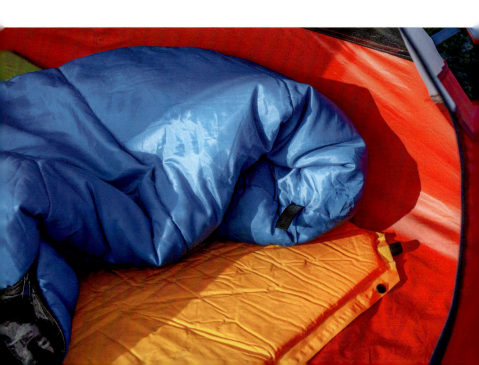

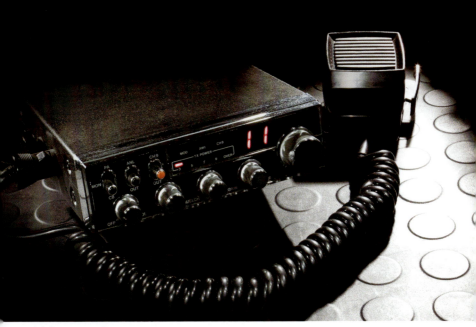

High frequency radio

Technology

Communication Technology

The Canadian hinterland is remote and vast in size with few roads and settlements and spotty cell phone coverage. Medical assistance could be hours away, so in the case of an emergency, you must have a means of communicating with proper authorities for assistance. The Royal Canadian Mounted Police are generally the first point of contact in the case of an emergency and often the first responders.

If you're going to be in a remote area for an extended period of time, it is a good idea to establish lines of communication based on a "sked," which is a schedule with set check-in times that you share with a chosen contact.

High Frequency and Very High Frequency Radios

When I worked in remote areas in northern Alberta, I relied on commercial grade High Frequency (HF) and Very High Frequency (VHF) radios to communicate with officials in the Alberta Forest Service based on a mutually agreeable sked. While

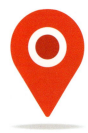

A word about troubleshooting portable devices used in vehicles: If it isn't working, check the fuse in both the car's electrical socket and the GPS power cable.

it wasn't always possible to get in touch with officials in Fort McMurray, the headquarters for the Athabasca Forest, or the town of Slave Lake, headquarters for the Slave Lake Forest, a towerman somewhere in these forests, could always relay messages. Both HF and VHF radios worked remarkably well, often over hundreds of miles.

HF is the designation for the range of radio frequency electromagnetic waves (radio waves) between 3 and 30 megahertz (MHz). The HF band is a major part of the shortwave band of frequencies, so communication at these frequencies is often called shortwave radio, popular with amateur (ham) radio buffs. These frequencies are suitable for long-distance communication and for mountainous terrains, which prevent line-of-sight communications.

The HF radios I used had a wire cable attached to the transmitter which could be strung high in a tree to receive a signal. The VHF radios had a built-in antenna. Both radios worked off batteries and were almost always reliable. VHF operates at a higher frequency range than HF, usually between 30–300 MHz. These transmissions, due to their higher frequency, penetrate through the ionosphere, with little or no refraction. VHF propagation is line-of-sight in nature and so is restricted to shorter-range communications.

There's no reason why you couldn't set up HF communications if you're in a remote area, provided you can find someone to engage with who is also equipped with a ham radio, out of a base camp of sorts, for example. On the other hand, handheld VHF 2-way radios would generally be suitable for communications between members of a party while in the outdoors.

I don't leave home without a 2-way radio nowadays; they're that important. There are many commercial brands of handheld radios with a long list of useful features on the market. I purchased Uniden handheld, 2-way radios several years ago to stay in touch with my outdoor partner(s). This brand features a lightweight, palm-sized radio you can clip on almost anywhere for ease of operating. It has 14 channels, up to 2-mile range, backlit display, clip-on design, 50 hours of operation (typical), low battery alert, call tone transmission and channel scan features. I recently purchased two sets of Motorola TALKABOUT radios because they feature an even greater range than the Uniden brand.

Satellite phones

Satellite phones have been on the market for several years. They work just about anywhere on the planet because they don't rely on a terrestrial cell phone network. Instead, they beam their data directly to and from satellites orbiting earth.

During a trip to the Upper Toobally Lake, Yukon—a remote, fly-in lake east of Watson Lake—my party rented a satellite phone in case of an emergency. They're expensive to purchase, but it only cost us $130 per week (plus GST) to rent, which we thought was a small price to pay. Before we departed, we made a list of emergency phone numbers in Yukon, so we knew who to call for help. Costs associated with voice calls from a satellite phone will vary anywhere from around $0.15 to

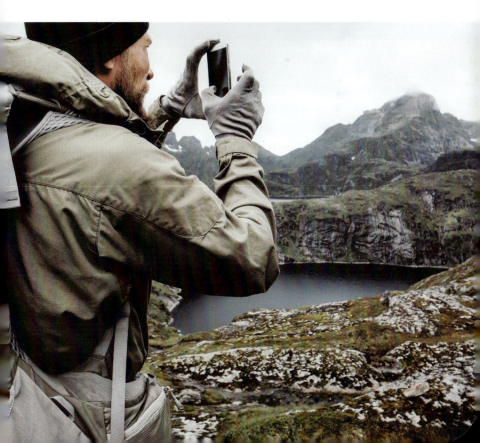

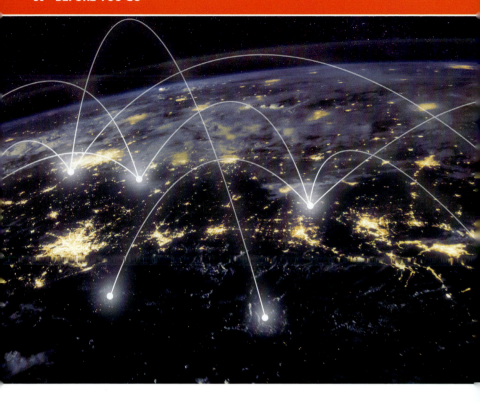

$2 per minute, with typical rates being from $0.80 to $1.50 per minute. Some providers will offer better rates within specific geographic areas. Our provider did not charge us for any airtime or for email messages.

inReach® Global Satellite Technology

David O'Farrell, Yukon outdoorsman and trapper, highly recommends inReach units and says he "wouldn't be without one" in his travels.

With inReach satellite technology from Garmin and a satellite subscription, you can stay in touch globally. You can send and receive messages, navigate your route, track and share your journey and, if necessary, trigger an SOS to get emergency help from a 24/7 global monitoring center via a global satellite network.

All inReach-enabled Garmin products offer GPS navigation—ranging from compass and bearing capabilities to basic grid waypoint marking and breadcrumb trails to sophisticated on-map guidance with detailed topographic maps, altimeter/barometer/compass reference and more.

In case of emergency, the inReach product can trigger an interactive SOS message to GEOS, a global safety company, that features a professional

24/7 global monitoring center. Their trained staff are available to respond to your message, track your device and notify emergency responders in your area, giving you the peace of mind that help is on the way. GEOS advises that they will stay in touch with you and your emergency contacts until your situation is resolved.

SPOT X Communication Device

Outdoor Canada Hunting Editor, Ken Bailey, advises, "When backcountry hunting, consider bringing a satellite phone or a messaging-capable device, such as the SPOT X Satellite GPS Messenger."

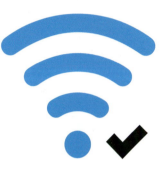

According to the company website, **SPOT X** provides 2-way satellite messaging when you're off the grid or beyond reliable cellular coverage. They advertise that you can connect SPOT X to your smart phone via Bluetooth wireless technology through the SPOT X app to access your contacts and communicate easily with family, friends or directly with Search & Rescue services in a life-threatening situation. Furthermore, if preferred or when necessary, SPOT X can be used as a stand-alone communication device. SPOT X has its own dedicated Canadian mobile number, so others can message you directly at any time.

Navigation Technology

A Global Positioning Receiver, called a GPS receiver, or simply GPS, is a device that is capable of receiving information from satellites that orbit the earth which calculate the device's (i.e., your) geographical position.

GPS systems are versatile and are used in many industrial sectors. They're optional equipment in most new vehicles, while portable units can also be plugged into electrical sockets to use as a navigational aid when driving.

A GPS system can help you to preplan your route and trace your route back home, so you should never get lost in the wild if the maps are up to date.

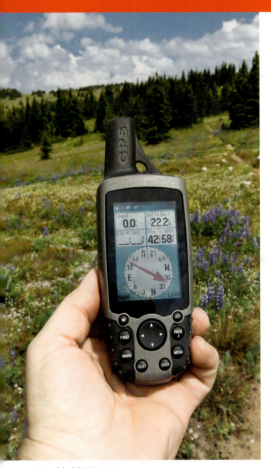

Hand-held GPS unit

Whether you use a GPS unit or your smartphone, ensure it is working properly, is charged or has new batteries and that you are otherwise prepared should your GPS fail.

Handheld units are also available for hikers. They can be used in airplanes on the ground or in the air. GPS systems are used by emergency crews to locate people in need of assistance. In theory, GPS receivers can work everywhere in the world, but in practice they are only useful in countries for which they have map data available. They provide you with locational information (i.e., "You are here") on a map display rather than meaningless raw latitude and longitude data. A GPS system can help you to preplan your route and trace your route back home, so you should never get lost in the wild if the maps are up to date.

Some GPS units feature an alarm so you can send a signal to alert your loved ones in case of danger from any location without cell service. They are not accurate, however, if maps used to program a GPS are not up to date and downloaded for the area that you'll be travelling in, and, if the batteries fail, they're useless. Further, in sub-zero weather—typical in Canadian winters—the batteries will not hold their charge. There's also a danger of losing a GPS unit. Some outdoorspeople are satisfied with apps on their smart phones, including the Google map application, and feel they're as good as a GPS unit.

Whether you use a GPS unit or your smartphone, ensure it is working properly, is charged or has new batteries and that you are otherwise prepared should your GPS fail.

Maps

Topographic (and Other) Maps

It is important that you understand how to read topographic (topo) and other maps, so you don't get lost! It is foolhardy to venture into unknown territory without having previously studied a topographic map of the area so you can chart your course safely. Topographic maps are available from various sources including map dealers, regional distribution centres, certified map printers and topographic map depositories.

Pay attention to the symbols in the Legend on your topographic map, especially with regard to hazards such as falls, rapids and contour intervals.

When I took basic training for the Canadian Army, and during my former various government jobs, it was essential to learn how to use topographic maps to perform my duties as a soldier, flight navigator, towerman, biologist and resource manager. Further, as a long-time angler and hunter, I routinely used topographic maps to chart travels in Canada's backcountry—likewise during time spent as a travel writer and outdoor journalist after I retired from my old day job(s). I have dozens of topographic maps that were essential to finding my way around the outdoors without getting lost. Similarly, I have what are called "recreational maps" of my favourite trails for Banff & Mount Assiniboine and Jasper & Maligne Lake in Alberta. I have maps of other favourite outdoor recreation areas, such as Kananaskis Country, Elk Island National Park, Waterton Lakes National Park and the Blackfoot Recreation Area. I take these maps and trail map brochures on my person when I travel

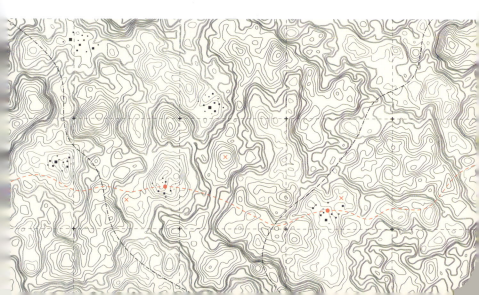

Before you head out, double check your maps so you know how long it will take to reach your destination after leaving the trailhead.

because they won't do me any good if they're at home. Before I head out, I double check the maps so I know how long it will take to reach my destination after leaving the trailhead. I also take notice of any cautionary notes that might require due diligence to avoid mishaps.

Note: Detailed, technical information related to Canada's topographic maps is available online (see Appendix) and is a valuable source of information for outdoors enthusiasts who plan to venture into unfamiliar territory.

Further, Canada's National Topographic System (NTS) map sheets offer detailed information on any particular area accurately and to scale. These maps depict in detail ground relief (landforms and terrain), drainage (lakes and rivers), forest cover, administrative areas, populated areas, transporta-

Take note of the symbols in the Legend on your topographic map, especially with regard to hazards such as falls and rapids and contour intervals.

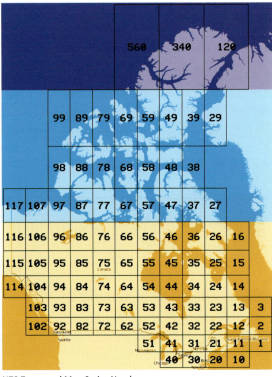

NTS Zones and Map Series Numbers
© OpenStreetMap contributors, CC BY-SA, CC BY-SA 2

tion routes and facilities (including roads and railways) and other human-made features. These maps are an excellent planning tool and guide that help make outdoor adventures enjoyable and safe.

A 1:50 000 scale topographic map is ideal for recreational activities. This scale accurately shows hills, valleys, lakes, rivers, streams, rapids, portages, trails, wooded areas, major, secondary and side roads, including all man-made features such as buildings, power lines, dams and cut lines. A 1:50 000 scale map covers an area approximately 1,000 square kilometres.

By comparison, a 1:250 000 scale topographic map is considered to be a reconnaissance-type map because it covers the same area of land as a sixteen (16) 1:50 000 scale map. This scale is useful as a detailed road map for driving on backroads and side roads. A full 1:250 000 scale map shows an area approximately the size of Prince Edward Island, Canada's smallest province.

A 1:50 000 scale topographic map is ideal for recreational activities.

Pay attention to the symbols in the Legend on your topographic map, especially with regard to hazards such as falls and rapids and contour intervals (marked in either "feet" or "metres") so you can estimate how much of a change in elevation is involved with trails, etc. by cross referencing contours with the map scale. Topographic maps can be plasticized so they're weatherproof, which will ensure the map lasts longer than a paper version when subjected to the elements.

Google Earth

In the absence of a topographic map, you can download map images of where you're going to be travelling from Google Earth on a smart phone or computer. Use the features on the map to guide you in deciding on a route by using a compass to keep your bearings. Key landmarks can be the waypoints: pipelines, power lines, lakes, streams, logged areas, roads, etc.

The Google Earth map will provide key topographic details of the area, while your compass will keep you going in the right direction if you plan your course according to the topography of the area. As a rule of thumb, most people walk about 5 kilometres per hour (or thereabouts), so you can estimate about how long it should take to travel from one point to another.

Most people walk about 5 kilometres per hour (or thereabouts), so you can estimate how long it should take to travel from one point to another.

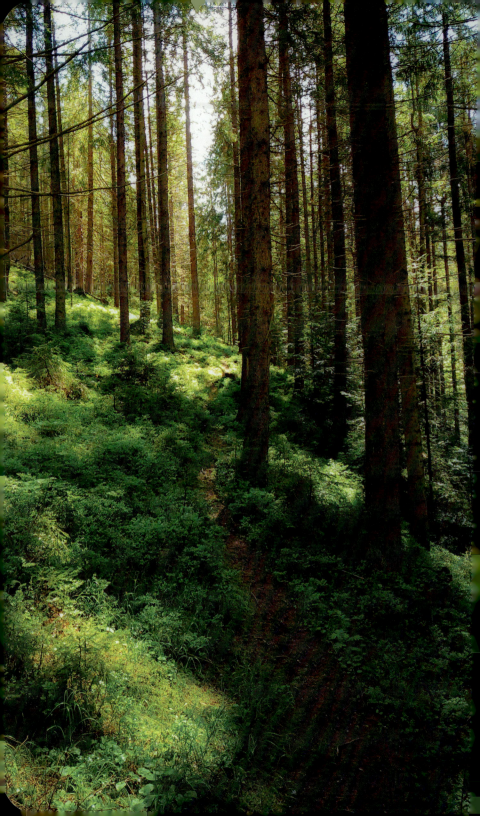

SECTION 2

In the Field: Survival Skills

>—⋊•⊙•⋉—<

If you don't know where you are going and it is safe to do so, stay put. Staying in one place can make is easier for search and rescue teams to find you.

Lore has it that people who are lost often end up traveling in circles, which is one reason why search and rescue teams suggest staying put to make it easier to find a lost person. If you're in a mountainous region, some say that you should follow a stream downstream, and you'll eventually find some sign of civilization. But if you don't actually know where you're going, you should just stay where you are.

This is probably the best and simplest advice. Transport Canada recommends that if you are in an aircraft that crashes in an uninhabited area, stay near the aircraft; their search is to locate the aircraft. If you are hiking or canoeing in a remote area and become stranded, the best advice is to remain where you are unless you are confident you can walk out on your own.

Always be prepared to spend time in the bush in case you do get lost, because this can happen to anyone. Wear appropriate footwear and clothing for the weather so you won't succumb to the elements. Build a makeshift shelter, gather enough wood for a campfire and do not waste time and energy on blind travel. Generally, your best option is to stay put if you do become disoriented until you can get your bearings and return to a trailhead.

The "STOP" Method

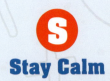

Stay Calm
Don't panic, get your breathing under control.

Trying to walk out when you don't know where you're going is foolhardy and not recommended by survival experts, especially in remote areas. If you are generally familiar with the area, you should use your common sense and follow the "STOP" method:

Think
Reconstruct your path back to the trailhead so you can figure out how to get back to where you started.

Look for a place that provides some emergency shelter, close to a source of wood for a campfire and, if possible, some water. If you are really lost, it is best that you simply stay put and focus on conserving your strength in the hopes that you will be found. If you have told other people about your plans, they can advise proper authorities to mount a search party.

Observe
Get hold of your bearings with a compass.

My advice in the event of an aircraft crash would be different: if you are not rescued after a week, you'll have to consider your circumstances and try to walk out to civilization.

Plan
Be careful to note landmarks as you head back to where you came from.

The "Survival Rule of Four"

The "Survival Rule of Four" addresses the basics of emergency survival essentials, as follows:

AIR	SHELTER	WATER	FOOD
4 MINUTES	4 HOURS	4 DAYS	4 WEEKS

You can survive **4 minutes** without **air**.

You can survive **4 hours** without **shelter**. (in harsh conditions)

You can survive **4 days** without **water**.

You can survive **4 weeks** without **food**.

The practicality of these rules must be taken into account relative to extreme survival situations. However, they are universally accepted as academic principles.

You must take immediate action regarding the first two principles (air and shelter), in particular, otherwise you will perish. In the case of the latter two principles, urgency is not as serious but still relevant in the longer term.

Fire

The Fire Triangle

The "fire triangle" illustrates the three elements a fire needs to burn. The triangle consists of oxygen in the air, heat generated by combustion and fuel such as firewood. It is with the combination of oxygen, heat and fuel that you start a fire "tetrahedron." Should you take any of these three things away, you either cannot start a fire or a fire will be extinguished. Try throwing a blanket on a fire and see what happens—in the absence of oxygen, the fire will go out. Without combustion from a match (heat), the fuel (firewood) will not burn, and if you run out of firewood, the fire will die. It's that simple.

Tinder

Tinder, which can be picked from the trunk of trees or from ground litter, works best to get the fire started.

Kindling

Kindling can be made by scraping an axe on the surface of dry wood or by using small twigs. The kindling should be placed on top of the tinder. Typically, I cut a large block of wood into small pieces and then chop these smaller pieces into thin slices as "kindling;" I also try to set some kindling aside to start a fire the next day.

IN THE FIELD • 91

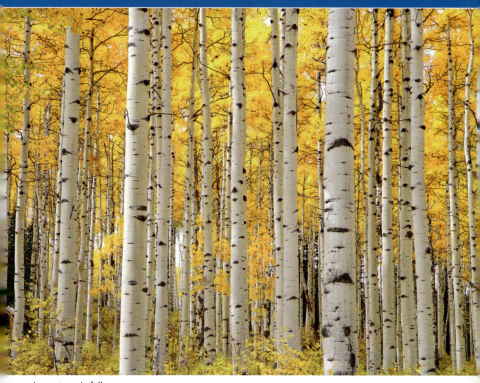

Aspen trees in fall

Softwood and Hardwood

In Canada, softwood comes from cottonwood, aspen popular or deciduous (evergreen) trees, whereas hardwood comes from the wood of birch or oak trees.

Softwood burns much faster than hardwood, so if you want to have some coals in the morning, it's a good idea to bank the fire with some hardwood. Some softwood like aspen popular burns very quickly, more so than deciduous trees.

Hardwood is ideal for cooking because it burns slower than softwood.

If you need to send a signal, any wood will work but softwood is easier to ignite and burns quickly as a signaling tool. Conifers also tend to give off more smoke it you want to be more visible.

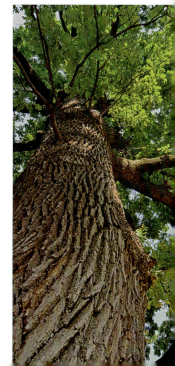

Oak tree

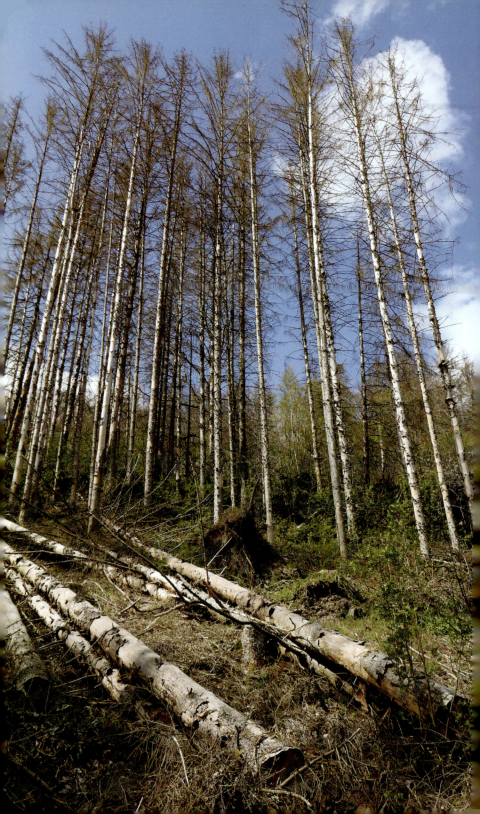

Wilderness Fire Locations

The best place to build a fire is a location that's out in the open and more likely to be fanned by a breeze so the smoke blows away. It should be built on level ground, scraped down to earth if possible. It should be surrounded by rocks and stones so the fire is contained and does not present a hazard. You don't want to start a forest fire so it should not be built close to combustible material. You should only build a fire that's large enough to cook on and provide some warmth or to dry out clothing, etc.

Finding Dry Firewood

Unless wood is dry it can be hard to cut with a saw or split with an axe.

Usually the best place to find dry firewood is on the edge of a clearing where trees tend to fall down due to winds if they suffer from rot or are old and decadent. Trees that are laying at an angle and not fully on the ground tend to be drier. You can also chop off the lower limbs on soft wood and hardwood trees which are the oldest branches and are suitable for firewood. In old burns there are usually lots of dead trees that are ideal for firewood. You can also find good firewood on the shores of lakes and banks of rivers where deadwood washes up, often in large log jams on rivers and streams.

Remember to pack some work gloves or leather gloves to protect your hands from splinters, cuts, bruises and burns.

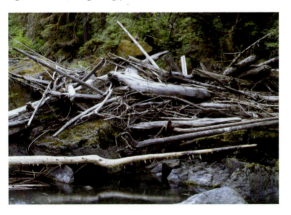

Usually the best place to find dry firewood is on the edge of a clearing where trees tend to fall down, or large log jams on rivers and streams.

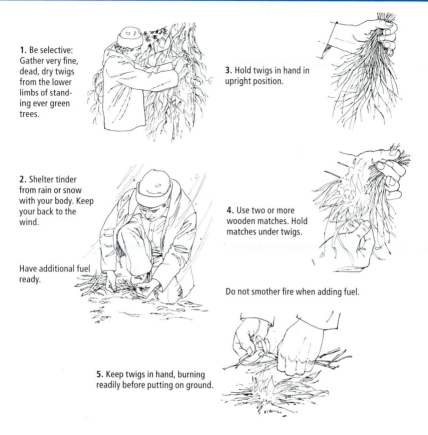

How to Start a Fire

Knowing how to build a fire is essential to outdoor survival. A fire can help a person stay warm under the most extreme cold weather; it can also be used to dry clothing, arrest hypothermia, signal for help during emergencies, cook food and stay safe and comfortable during the night. To light a fire, you will need matches, a steel striker or a butane lighter, of which there are many brands on the market.

The Fire Pit

It is best practice to build a fire pit before trying to start a fire. The fire pit should be in the open. You can set rocks and boulders in a circle or set a couple of logs side by side with some space in between each log. If the ground is dry, scrape the forest litter to the side so you don't start a forest fire by accident. During the winter, scrape snow off the ground before creating a fire pit so it won't put out a fire when it melts. If the snow is very deep, remove as much snow as possible and lay a bedding of branches in the fire pit.

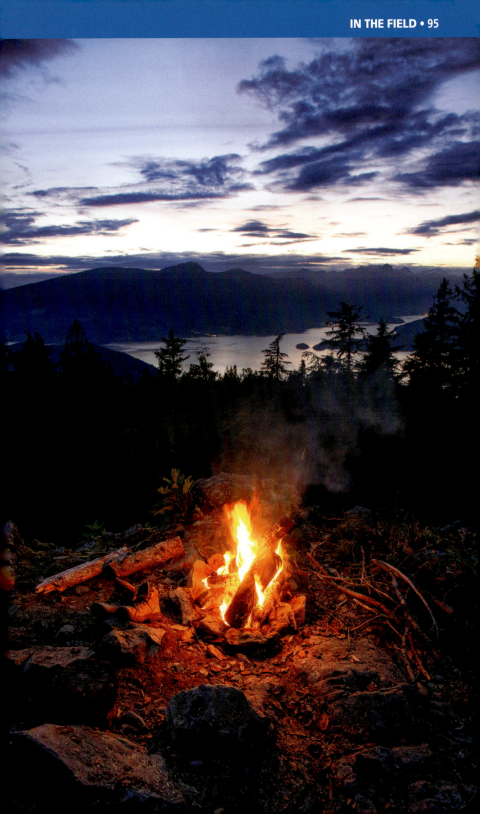

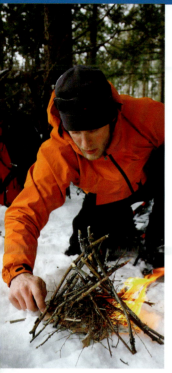

The Teepee Method

One of the easiest ways to build a fire is to pile wood the size of kindling first with larger logs on the outside in the shape of a pyramid. Lastly, top off the kindling using some larger branches, also fashioned in a pyramid shape, before setting the tinder on fire. Usually, this method works very well, especially if it's windy when the log cabin method might experience some issues.

The Log Cabin Method

The log cabin fire is another popular set-up for starting a campfire. It is also known as the "criss cross fire." It is essentially a criss-cross build of small to medium sized wood shaped in the form of cabin that can burn down to create a quick cooking fire. I believe it's a matter of personal preference whether to use the teepee method or log cabin method, but the former is my first choice for wilderness campfires.

Teepee method

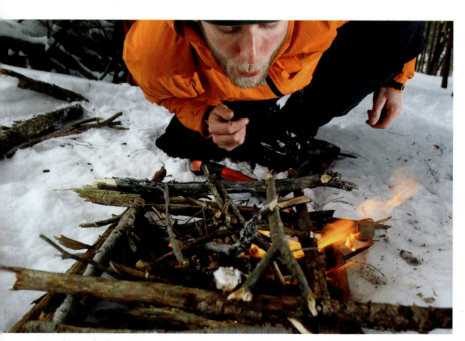

Log cabin method

Matches and Lighters (Waterproof)

Old fashioned wooden matches with sulfur heads date back to 1828 when they were patented in Britain. So long as they are dry, they are very reliable to start a campfire or ignite any combustible material. If they get wet the heads dissolve, and they won't work. Consequently, for wilderness travel I prefer to use waterproof and windproof matches, which are more expensive but fail-safe. However just to be on the safe side, before I ignite any tinder, I always use them in tandem, so if one fails to strike the other probably will.

Butane lighters remain popular but tend to flame out if there's any amount of wind, plus they often burn a person's fingers while trying to start a campfire, so matches are my preference. They're a good standby, however, so it doesn't hurt to carry one in your gear and use them if winds are calm.

Steel Wool & Battery Method

You can easily start a fire with a 9-volt battery and some steel wool (not a coarse grain, and the finer the grain the better) just by rubbing the battery terminals against the wool a few times. The wool will quickly start to spark. Use the sparks to light your tinder to get a fire started.

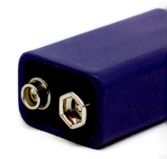

Flint & Steel Method

The benefit of using a flint and steel is that this method not affected by cold temperatures or poor weather. Strike the steel (repeatably) in an angled, downward direction against the flint toward a combustible material to create sparks to start a fire.

Magnifying Glass

In a pinch you could start a fire with a magnifying glass. Although this might not be very practical in much of Canada, it will work. Just shine the beam of light on some tinder and eventually it will create ignition. This method does not work if it's cloudy and works best on warm, sunny days. You need a small focal point to get a fire started.

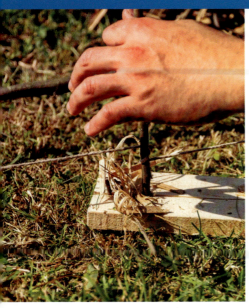

The Bow Drill

The bow drill works by spinning a piece of wood in the socket of another piece of wood. The friction creates a small coal that can with care be blown into a flame to ignite tinder. The bow drill can require a lot of time and effort before a good coal can be created. Use only dry wood for the spindle and fireboard for best results; green wood won't work. There are online videos that illustrate how to spin the spindle with a bow. Cottonwood, aspen, cedar or willow are likely the best woods in Canada to use for this method.

The Fire Plough

The fire plough (or fire plow) is a primitive tool used to light a fire. In its simplest form this amounts to using two sticks rubbed together. I've used this method and found it a very difficult procedure, but with effort it will work. The point of one piece of wood is rubbed quickly against the groove of a second piece in a "plowing" motion to produce hot dust that then becomes a coal. A split is often made down the length of the grooved piece, so that oxygen can flow freely to the coal or ember to aid the ignition process.

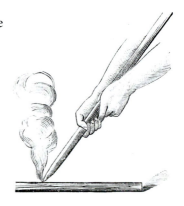

The Hand Drill

A hand drill is another, simpler version of the bow drill where a hand held stick is rubbed against a (flat) piece of wood to create friction and ignite a spark to create a flame and start a fire. The hand drill method of friction fire making is about as primitive as it gets. You spin a wooden drill against a wood board with your bare hands. This method is reported as having one of the widest distributions on earth, and it probably has been used for the longest span of time.

Accelerants

In adverse conditions, some commercial fire starter will help get a fire started. You can also use lighter fluid, gasoline or aerosol sprays for the same purpose. If you hold a match in front of an aerosol spray it will create a combustion torch.

Dryer Lint

A cheap, reliable fire starter (i.e., tinder) is lint from your dryer, which contains all manner of highly combustible material. Use two or three matches held together to set the tinder ablaze.

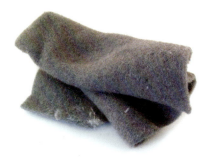

Wax & Fibre

Wax (i.e., paraffin) is highly combustible when combined with fibre (e.g., cotton balls or rags) and together they can be an effective accelerant. If conditions are wet, wax and fibre will help get a fire started quickly.

Hand Sanitizer & Gauze Pad

Hand sanitizer is made of alcohol which if highly flammable. Soak some gauze with hand sanitizer to create a cheap, simple accelerant that will create instant ignition when lighted.

Cotton Ball & Petroleum Jelly

Petroleum jelly is a hydrocarbon that is flammable and when squeezed into cotton balls is a good DIY accelerant that's affordable and easy to make. Store the cotton balls in a small Ziploc bag.

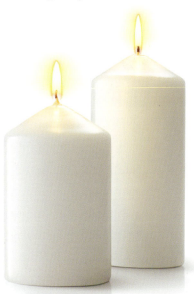

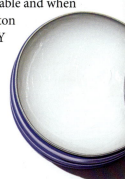

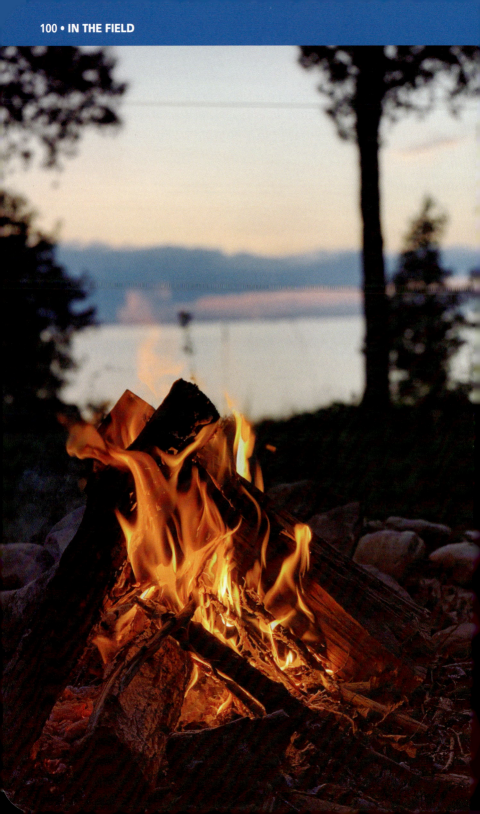

Proper Placement of Fire

Follow guidelines elsewhere in this book regarding the proper placement of fire so you don't accidentally start a forest fire and to ensure you get your best bang for your buck for both cooking and heating.

Fire Tending

You'll need a large supply of firewood to make it through the night. The firewood should be within easy reach. It's also a good idea to keep some kindling in reserve to help re-start a fire should it die out.

Construct a Camp Stove

The best camp stoves are commercial products. (Coleman has long been an industry leader with its white gas, portable, functional stove(s) that also runs on propane.) You can however create a simple camp stove by building a rock crib with a steel grill on top of it over a fire. Such DIY stoves work best once the firewood has burned down so cooking is done over the more even heat provided by coals, not wood that has just been ignited and tends to flare.

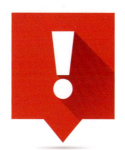

Fire Safety

A word of caution: It is absolutely essential to put out fires when you break camp. Under no circumstances should a fire be left burning because it can cause a forest fire. Douse it with water to ensure there are no flames or burning embers before you leave.

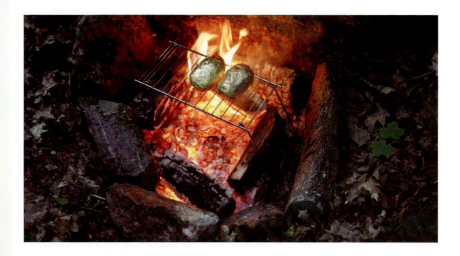

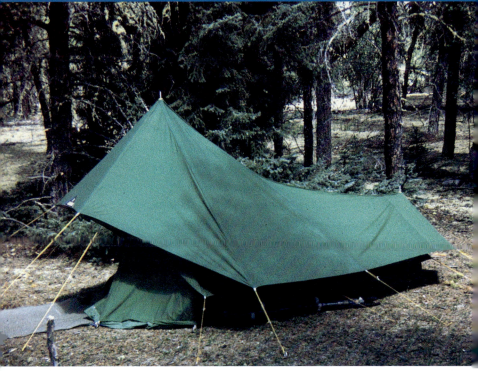

Never cook or store food in your sleeping tent.

Shelter

Location

It is important to select a suitable location for your campsite or shelter when you are in the bush. There should be a source of firewood if you plan to use fire to stay warm or cook meals. The location where you plan to pitch your tent should be on a level spot that's well drained; if you don't pitch your tent on level ground, you'll be rolling around all night and will not sleep well, and there is nothing worse than having water seep into your tent during a rainstorm, especially because it can be hard to dry things out afterward. Clear the site of rocks and roots.

Further, you want to be above the high-water mark if you're camping beside a stream or lake. You'd be surprised how high waves can get along a beach following a windstorm. R.M. Patterson (*The Dangerous River*) describes an event beside the Nahanni River in the Northwest Territories in which the river rose 6-7 feet in an hour!

If possible, a location that is exposed to prevailing winds is ideal to keep pesky mosquitoes and black flies at bay. Black flies lay their eggs in streams, particularly near the outlets, and their larvae attach to the substrate until they hatch. These places are to be avoided during the summer because some hatches can be spread out over several weeks and there could be plagues of black flies.

Be wary of pitching a camp near a game trail, especially if you're unarmed, because you never know what might show up. Bears, cougars and wolves all follow game trails, and it's best to avoid encounters with them. Trail camera footage illustrates just how often large carnivores such as grizzly and black bears, cougars and wolves travel along game trails at night. If also best to stay away from streams, where the sound of water can drown out other sounds, including approaching animals or potential rescuers.

Keeping a Clean Campsite

It is key to keep your campsite clean at all times. Under no circumstances should you keep any food in a tent when in bear country or cook inside a tent; this is verboten. Bring an extra tent for cooking if necessary. There are anecdotal stories that grizzlies can smell a dead carcass from several miles away, so you can well imagine they'd pick up the scent of bacon being cooked over a campfire, leading the bear to where you're camping.

Food should be stored away from your campsite, best hung in a tree out of reach of bears, and it's a good idea to clean all cooking utensils, pots and pans so they do not attract unwanted animals to your campsite. For the same reason, you should not sleep in clothes that you've cooked in as the odor will stay in this clothing.

Toilet functions should be performed away from your campsite, so they don't attract bears. Human waste should be buried and covered with dirt for the same reason.

Food should be stored away from your campsite, best hung in a tree out of reach of bears, and it's a good idea to clean all cooking utensils, pots and pans so they do not attract unwanted animals to your campsite.

Building a Shelter

The shelter should protect you from the elements and keep you dry to prevent the loss of body heat. Pick a site that allows you to build a fire in front of it, so the heat is reflected into the shelter.

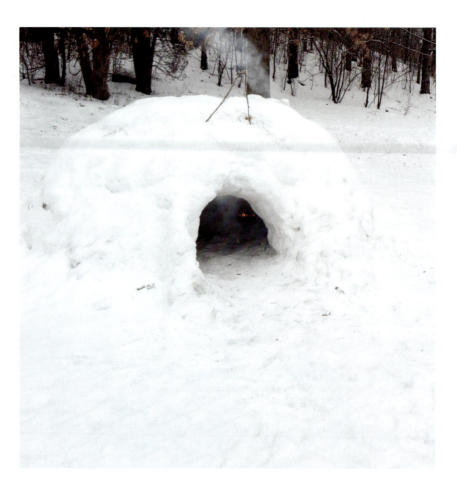

Quinzee Hut

A quinzhee, or quinzee, is a Canadian snow hut or shelter that is made from a large pile of loose snow, shaped into a low-lying dome and then hollowed out to provide shelter from the elements. In my opinion, this is a last resort type of shelter for reasons explained elsewhere in this book. The idea is to make a snow pile that's large enough to make a cave inside it, using whatever tools you have available, or by hand if necessary. Afterward, create a hollow to lie in out of the elements, with adequate space to breathe.

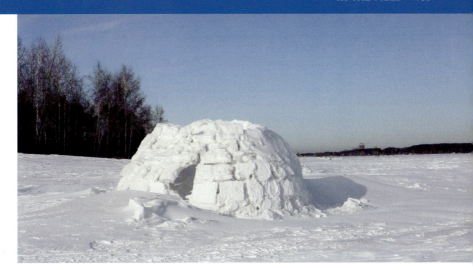

Igloo

An igloo is built up from blocks of hard snow and is a traditional shelter built by the Inuit. It would be impossible for most people to build an igloo without proper tools or training. For these reasons it's best to use other portable shelters that are easier, quicker and more practical, such as nylon tents.

Snow Cave

A snow cave is constructed by digging into a snowbank made up of compacted, relatively hard drifted snow. In many parts of Canada, it would be possible to use snow caves as emergency shelters because prevailing winds often create huge snow drifts. It's simple and straightforward to use a shovel to create an opening in such drifts that would be the entrance to a larger opening further inside the drift. As a kid growing up in the Crowsnest Pass, I'd often construct such snow caves with my friends. The snow was packed so it was safe, but there is always the danger of a cave in so they should be built with caution and used as a last resort.

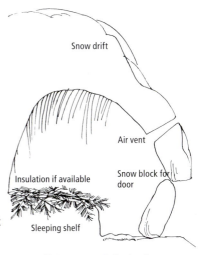

Not recommended unless in area where no other type of shelter can be made.

Tarp Structures (Hammock, Wraps)

Some outdoors people opt for tarps to provide overnight shelters, not so much a hammock or wrap in Canada which I would view as a liability. Tarps come in various sizes (i.e., 10' x 12' - 12' x 20' - 12' x 30' - 14' x 20' - 18' x 20' - 20' x 20', etc.). They are usually made of canvas or plastic such as polyethylene so they're waterproof and windproof. They have gromets on the corners so they can be secured with a rope to a make shift ridge poles tied between a couple of trees. I believe that tarps should be standard outdoor gear and I always carry at least one on any wilderness trip.

Forester's Tent

A forester's tent is set up using three wooden poles—two of which are the same length, set up in an A-frame at the front of what will become the tent, and a longer ridge pole that slopes toward the rear of the tent, extends to the front and is positioned on top of the two front poles. A tarp can be set up over top of the ridge pole and tied to the poles that make up the A-frame. Aluminum pegs can be used to hold down the sides of the tarp. You can switch the front for the back simply by re-positioning the ridge pole if a wind comes up. A campfire built in front of the tent will provide enough heat to stay warm even in extremely cold weather.

Lean-to Tent

With a tarp, you can also make a lean-to tent. The tarp is hung over a ridge pole that is positioned on top of two poles at either end that have been erected in the style of an A-frame and tied together with twine or a cable tie at the top.

The lean-to tent should be pitched at an angle from the front to the back and will provide shelter for a person and their bedding and gear. With a campfire at the front it will be warm and comfortable, especially if built in a sheltered, treed area.

For some types of emergency shelters, you will need an axe or hatchet (see section **Axes, Hatchets and Saws** on page 67).

Lean-to Shelter

A lean-to shelter is one of the most basic and easiest of shelters to build in forested areas. Select a suitable spot on level ground and between two trees where you can set up a ridge pole between them that is several feet apart. The ridge pole can be supported by a forked stick or laid on top of a notch provided by a tree branch on the trunk of a tree. You can also use some parachute cord to tie the ridge pole to a tree trunk. Next, cut several framing poles and spread them about 12 inches apart along the ridge pole, at an angle, facing backward so that most of the weight is up against the trunks of the two trees. Thatch evergreen boughs between the framing poles of the lean-to shelter. Finish by fashioning a bed of evergreen boughs at least several inches deep to provide good insulation from the cold ground under the shelter.

Keep in mind that in sub-zero temperature, the temperature at ground level will be about zero, but that is still warmer than ambient temperatures. Make a fire pit in front of the lean-to shelter. A simple fire pit can be made between two large trees cut into pieces about three to four feet in length. Tinder can be placed under some kindling to get the fire going, which can then be fed with larger firewood.

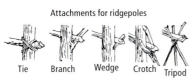

Attachments for ridgepoles

Tie   Branch   Wedge   Crotch   Tripod

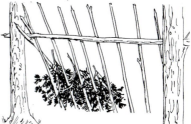

3. Start with largest boughs at the bottom with butt ends up.

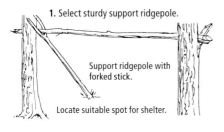

1. Select sturdy support ridgepole.

Support ridgepole with forked stick.

Locate suitable spot for shelter.

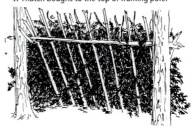

4. Thatch boughs to the top of framing pole.

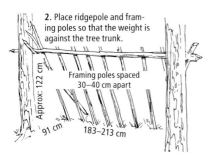

2. Place ridgepole and framing poles so that the weight is against the tree trunk.

Framing poles spaced 30–40 cm apart

Approx: 122 cm

91 cm   183–213 cm

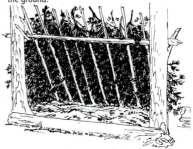

5. A bough bed will insulate you from the ground. Boughs should be placed with broken ends toward the ground.

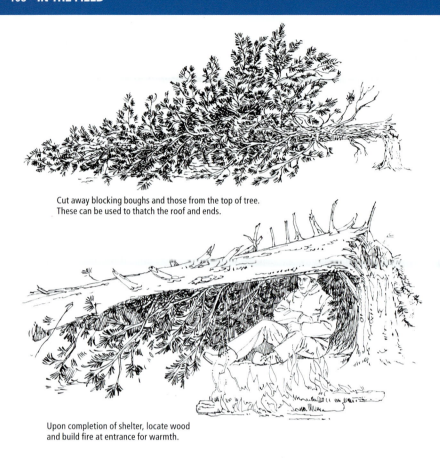

Cut away blocking boughs and those from the top of tree. These can be used to thatch the roof and ends.

Upon completion of shelter, locate wood and build fire at entrance for warmth.

Fallen Tree Shelter

If you're in a forested area, search out a fallen evergreen tree that has enough space between it and the ground to move around safely. Use an axe or hatchet to cut off some branches along the top and sides of the tree, which should then be leaned against the trunk to make a roof. The backside of the shelter can function as a windbreak. Obviously, you don't want to cut off any of the branches that might be supporting the tree. Once the shelter has been completed, build a fire pit at the entrance for warmth.

Leaf Structure

A leaf structure shelter is one of the most basic and primitive emergency shelters. It is normally made for a single person from branches, fallen leaves and forest litter. Start by selecting a stout branch that can be used as a spine (i.e., a tree branch that exceeds your height and is free of limbs) as a main support for the structure. Next, you'll need two load bearing tree branches that can be joined together to support the spine. If you can, use branches with forked ends to eliminate the need that they be lashed together with twine. Put the spine at the apex of the two load bearing trees in the shape of an elongated tripod. Afterward, lay smaller tree branches on either side of the spine and keep adding tree branches until you've created a wall of sorts. Finally, put fallen leaves on top of these branches to cover the walls of the shelter. It won't be pretty, but if done carefully, you'll have shelter from the elements.

Bough Bed

A bough bed is not a shelter, per se. Rather it is a mattress made of logs and evergreen branches that probably had its genesis in the Canadian fur trade. The main benefit of a bough bed would be in cold weather to keep your body off the ground to ensure your body heat loss is minimized. You would have to build it inside a larger shelter. An axe or bow saw would help when constructing a bough bed. You'll need the following material:

- Several branches from evergreen trees, such as fir that feature soft needles
- Four logs that are longer than you are tall
- Four logs that are approximately 3 feet long
- Several feet of twine or rope
- Saplings to span the length of the bedframe

Lay out two of the long logs about three feet apart and form a crib with two of the shorter logs placed at either end. Repeat the process with the remaining logs so you have what amounts to a bed frame, laying the remaining logs across the frame to make it sturdy. Tie the logs on the corners with some twine so they don't move. Lay ½ inch saplings lengthwise over the cross beams. Finally, use the evergreen tree branches to make what amounts to a mattress by laying them crosswise on top of the saplings.

Natural Shelters and Caves

A cave or rock outcrop are obvious sites to spend the night. Be wary of these places because they may harbour predators such as cougars and especially bears overwinter. They may also be used by bats, which may carry rabies. Some caves might also be used as hibernacula for poisonous snakes that use them as overwinter dens. Other forms of wildlife such as bighorn sheep will also seek refuge in caves during inclement weather.

Use your common sense when selecting caves or outcrops as shelters. If there are animal scats, droppings, fur or hair nearby you should be wary. These are signs of potential danger. Be on guard.

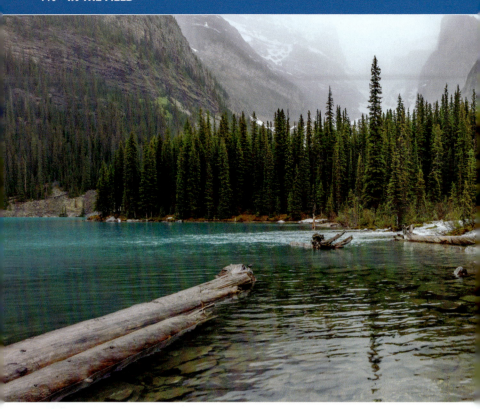

Water

Drinking water

Water is a key element in outdoor survival, as necessary as food and shelter. It is vital that you stay hydrated to maintain your balance and orientation as well as to prevent both mental and physical fatigue. You should hydrate yourself with about a litre of water before you start hiking. If you become dehydrated, you can develop a headache and get dizzy. Take enough water to get through the day or a filter to purify water along the trail. Sip water during your hike; don't drink it in bilges, which your body won't store. If it's going to be very hot, you can expect to go through a litre of water each hour. The amount of water you'll need varies from person to person and according to the length and difficulty of the trial and weather conditions.

That being said, you can't be too careful when sourcing drinking water, regardless of where you are in Canada's outdoors. Water might not be suitable for human consumptions for a variety of reasons, even in what might look like pristine conditions. Water can be very alkaline or saline, it may contain

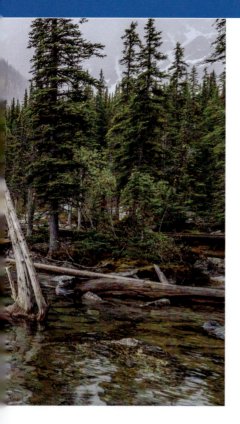

toxic contaminants (e.g., hydrocarbons, herbicides or pesticides), toxic blue green algae, fecal coliform material or water borne parasites.

Often, you will need a device that that filters and purifies water by removing bacteria, protozoa, viruses and suspended solids. (There are also many brands of water purification tablets.)

My first experience with dirty water in Canada's north country happened when I was doing biological surveys on tributary streams to the mighty Peace River. If you took a bucket of water from the river, you couldn't see the bottom. After the sediment settled, it was still unfit to drink, so we had to source cooking and drinking water from a nearby river that was flowing clear. Generally, I boil water in a large pot after dinner to be used for cooking and drinking water the next day. I didn't get sick once over the course of four long summers in the bush of the boreal forest in northern Alberta.

Tannins in water from ubiquitous acidic muskeg bogs in Canada's boreal forest can cause chronic migraine headaches in some people. The most severe sufferers of tannin sensitivity can have joint pain that mimics arthritis, fatigue, depression, digestive problems, vision problems, attention deficit, thin, brittle skin, eczema, acid reflux and heartburn, dizziness, headaches, racing heart, slowed metabolism, hair loss, multiple chemical sensitivity, muscle weakness, jitteriness, panic attacks, insomnia, flash fevers (toxic flushes), susceptibility to colds, gastrointestinal disorders and other ailments due to nutrients in food not being absorbed wholly or efficiently into the bloodstream.

Generally speaking, water that flows from a spring will be safe to drink but be cautious when drinking water from other sources. It's a good idea to boil, filter or purify water if in doubt.

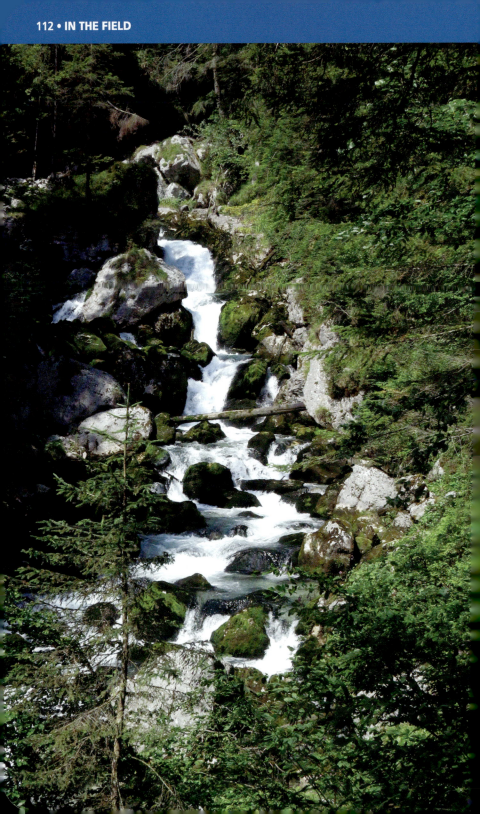

Finding Water

Head Downhill

Water is subject to gravity, so it always flows downhill. If you're looking for water in upland areas and can't find any, then head to lower elevations where it might be ponded or surface at springs in hillsides. Water is generally locally abundant across most of Canada and is ubiquitous in the northern territories, but there are many arid areas—especially in the western provinces—where it can be scarce. Never take it for granted that water will be present, because in addition to the foregoing it is not unusual for periodic droughts to occur, especially in western Canada.

Vegetation Moisture

Moisture tends to collect on grasses and leaves overnight as temperature cool. It can be wiped or licked off grass and leaves as a source of drinking water. Likewise, moisture also accumulates on tents and tarps during the summer—another source of drinking water.

Freshwater Springs

Freshwater springs are a good source of drinking water and, as a rule, should be safe to drink. Water that percolates out of the ground through sand and gravel is generally free of contaminants. Look for springs on the lower levels of hillsides and especially cutbanks.

> **If you're looking for water in upland areas and can't find any, then head to lower elevations where it might be ponded or surface at springs in hillsides.**

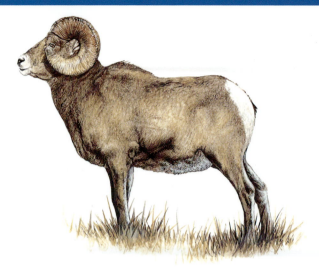

Animal Tracks and Trails

Animals need water to survive, and some will travel a considerable distance each day for a daily drink. Look for animal tracks and game trails that will often lead to sources of water. Some animals such as bighorn sheep may travel a mile or more each evening to a source of water.

Rainwater

Rainwater can be collected if you have a tarp or plastic sheet to catch it and funnel it into a container.

Ice and Snow

Ice and snow are ideal sources of water but they must be melted before they release water, so you'll need a pot and fire to obtain water from either of them.

Digging

Water seeps into the ground and becomes "groundwater," which can be located by digging a hole in the ground in areas that are most likely be close to the surface. The presence of vegetation usually is a sign that water is nearby.

Streams and Lakes

Streams and lakes are the most reliable sources of water, but be careful of muskeg drained areas which may cause some digestive problems (see below for further details).

Morning Dew

Morning dew is the water droplets we find in the morning on leaves and other objects outside, and usually in spring or winter when the air is cold. Dew is similar to rain because it forms from water vapour.

Water Purification and Filtration

Solar Still

If you have a piece of plastic and a container to store water, you can collect and purify water in the backcountry by using a solar still. Solar stills are a device originally designed for army and navy fliers forced down in the oceans that converts salt water or contaminated water into drinking water by vaporization by the sun's rays and condensation. By definition, a solar still is a simple distillation device consisting of a sheet of plastic placed over a pit, allowing water vapour produced by evaporation to run back into a collection vessel. A solar still distills water with substances dissolved in it by using the heat of the sun to evaporate water so that it may be cooled and collected free from substances or contaminates, thereby purifying it.

Don't expect to find clean drinking water in the outdoors. Be sure to bring plenty of water with you and/or a water filter or purifier.

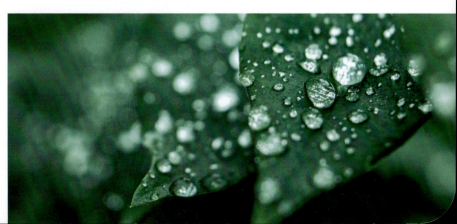

Giardia

Giardia duodenalis, also known as *Giardia intestinalis* and *Giardia lamblia*, is a waterborne parasitic microorganism that colonizes and reproduces in the small intestine, causing a diarrheal condition known as giardiasis. It can be picked up by hikers or campers who drink untreated water from springs, lakes, or rivers. Typical symptoms include an upset stomach, cramps and often severe diarrhea. When it was first diagnosed in Canada it was called "beaver fever." Symptoms may last for two to six weeks if left untreated and manifest one to two weeks after a person becomes infected. Many prescription drugs are available to treat giardiasis.

Purification versus Filtration

Water purification is the process of removing undesirable chemicals, biological contaminants, suspended solids and gases from untreated water to produce water that is suitable for a specific purpose, such as drinking water. On the other hand, water filtration is the process of separating suspended solid matter such as particles, parasites, bacteria, algae, viruses and fungi from a liquid by causing the latter to pass through the pores of some substance called a filter. The liquid which has passed through the filter is called the filtrate.

Giardia duodenalis

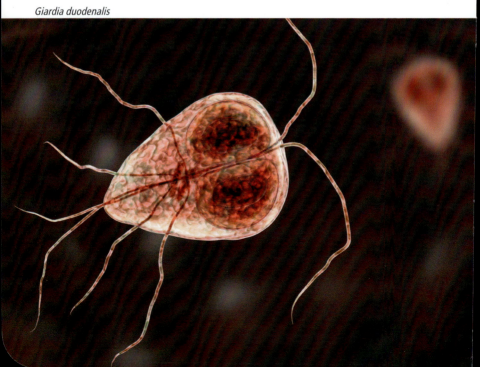

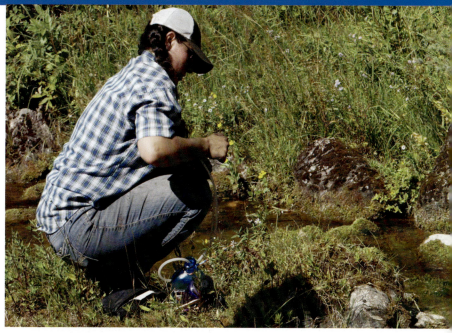
Use a water purifyer in the bush.

For brevity, purification removes invisible contaminants while filtration removes visible contaminants. There are several techniques used to either purify or filter water so it's safe to drink described as follows.

Boiling Water

If you do not have bottled water, you should boil water from a lake or stream to ensure that it's safe to drink. Boiling will kill harmful bacteria, viruses and waterborne protozoa such as giardia. If water is cloudy with silt, let it settle and then filter it through a clean cloth, paper towel or a large coffee filter.

Bring water to a rolling boil for at least one minute. Boiling bottles for five minutes will sterilize them.

A word of caution, some water is so heavily laden with sediment it may have to be filtered several times to remove particulate matter before it can be boiled.

Purification removes invisible contaminants while filtration removes visible contaminants.

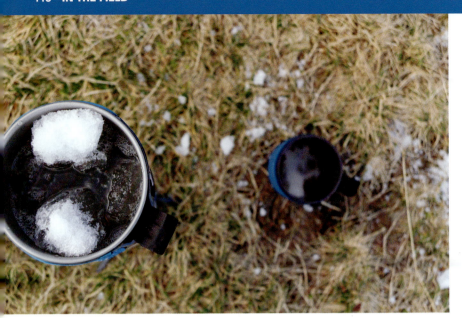

Melting Snow

During the winter when lakes and streams are frozen, you may have to melt snow in a pot as a source of drinking water. Fill the pot to the brim with snow and put it over a fire to melt, adding additional snow as the first batch melts until the pot is nearly full of water. As a rule of thumb, bring water to a rolling boil for 1 minute; if you're above 6,500 feet, boil it for 3 minutes to purify it.

DIY Rock and Sand Filter

If you don't have the means to boil your water, you can make a DIY rock and sand filter as a primitive filtration system. Use a large plastic milk or soda pop container as a makeshift filter by cutting off the bottom and turning it upside down so it can function as a funnel. Put a cloth in the bottom of the container (near the neck) and add layers of rock and sand on top of the cloth. Pour water through the funnel into a container to filter out sediment.

Charcoal Filter

A charcoal filter can be made the same way as a DIY rock and sand filter simply by substituting activated carbon (i.e., refined charcoal) for the rock and sand. Activated charcoal can be obtained from retail outlets.

A word of caution: activated carbon filters will not remove microbial contaminants such as bacteria and viruses, calcium and magnesium (hard water minerals), fluoride, nitrate and many other compounds.

Iodine Tablets

Online sources indicate that iodine used for water purification is commonly added to water as a solution, in crystallized form, or in tablets containing tetraglycine hydroperiodide that release 8 mg of iodine per tablet. Iodine can be added to untreated water to kill harmful microorganisms and make the water safer to drink. The iodine kills many, but not all, of the most common pathogens present in natural fresh water sources.

Chlorine Dioxide Tablets

Chlorine dioxide is a very effective bacterial disinfectant, and it is even more effective than chlorine for the disinfection of water that contains viruses. Chlorine dioxide is mainly used as a bleach in the paper industry and for the treatment of drinking water. Because of its unique qualities, it is effective as a disinfectant against viruses, bacteria, and parasitic cysts, such as giardia even at low concentrations.

Chlorine dioxide is available in tablets. Manufacturers claim that it requires a 4-hour treatment time for effectiveness.

Potassium Permanganate

Potassium permanganate is a strong oxidizing agent with some disinfectant properties. It was used extensively before hypochlorites as a drinking water disinfectant. It is most commonly used as a 1–5 percent solution for disinfection and often sold as packets of 1 gram to be added to 1 litre of water. Potassium permanganate is marketed as a point-of-entry treatment option for water, sold as a dry, purple-tinted solid. It oxidizes dissolved particles of iron, hydrogen sulfide, and manganese so that the solid particles can be easily filtered out of water. The chemical will give treated water a pink colour.

The LifeStraw

The "LifeStraw" is a brand that manufactures water filtration and purification devices. The first product was designed as a portable water filter "straw." Manufacturers claim that it filters a maximum of 4000 litres of water—enough for one person for three years—and removes almost all waterborne bacteria, microplastics and parasites. LifeStraw uses an advanced, special formulation that is made from fibres, instead of traditional granulated carbon, which improves longevity and performance. The filtration process works via adsorption—contaminants become trapped inside the pore structure of the carbon and bind to the surfaces.

Food: Foraging, Trapping and Fishing

Foraging: Rules and Tips

Safety

Canada has a wide variety of plants that can provide us with food, clothing, medicine and shelter. There are several Canadian field guides that provide information on this subject. One of the most comprehensive guides is *Edible & Medicinal Plants of Canada* (2014) (see Appendix on page 250). The key advice from this guide is to never gather plants unless you are sure of their identity because some plants are poisonous or can cause allergic reactions. Use a plant field guide to get familiar with the local species you may encounter as you venture through the Canada's backcountry.

WARNING: Never gather plants unless you are sure of their identity because some plants are poisonous or can cause allergic reactions.

I will summarize below key wild (or feral) edible plants for short term survival only. "Garden" variety plants are another story, such as daffodils, giant hogweed, winterberry, American nightshade and American pokeweed, all of which are poisonous. Some edible plants, such as elderberry berries, should not be eaten raw, used only in jams and pies. In fact, the berries of many wild plants that have been used to make jams and jellies aren't a good food source for short-term survival. Other examples include rosehips, whose outer, fleshy part can be eaten, but the inner seeds are not palatable and can cause digestive issues. Likewise, the seed in cherries contain cyanide and are poisonous, and northern black currants can cause severe diarrhea and vomiting unless mixed with cranberries—in fact, eating large quantities of any berries can cause diarrhea. As a rule, be careful eating berries that you cannot accurately identify.

Remember, you can do without food for about a week, so you won't starve to death in the short term. Canada has sophisticated search and rescue teams, so should you get lost, you will hopefully be found alive and well in short order. However, it is important to eat to maintain your strength. The following list will focus on short-term food coping requirements:

Edible Plants

Asparagus

Asparagus grows in the wild in every province in Canada, especially in moist areas nears lakes and streams, and is usually found in patches. The plant grows in bunches. It is not a "wild" plant, per se, and would be classified as being feral.

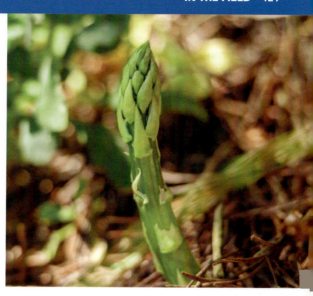

Blackberries, Raspberries and Cloudberry

Blackberries, raspberries and cloudberry are all related to each other. Both blackberries and raspberries can be eaten fresh. Blackberries can be stored (usually dried) for use in the winter. Only the berries of blackberry and raspberry bushes should be eaten as the wilted leaves can be toxic. Cloudberry berries have twice the concentration of vitamin C as an orange.

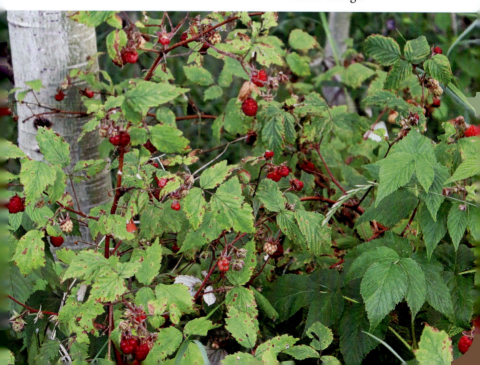

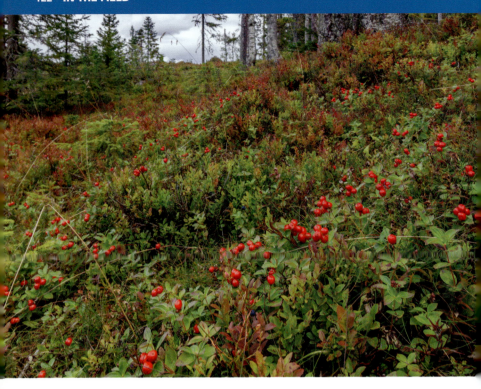

Bearberries or Kinnikinnick

While bearberries are mealy and tasteless, they are usually abundant and remain on branches of the bearberry or kinnikinnick evergreen shrub year-round, so they can be an important survival food. However, too many bearberries can cause constipation. The kinnikinnick plant is common throughout much of Canada, especially in wet areas.

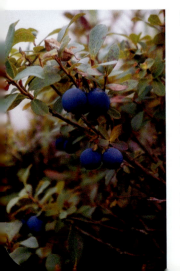

Blueberries and Huckleberries

The round purplish berries of huckleberries resemble blueberries, and in some parts of North America, huckleberries are called blueberries, though they are not the same fruit. Huckleberries are found only in montane areas of Alberta and British Columbia, while blueberries are present in all provinces in Canada. Both huckleberries and blueberries are abundant in the late summer and autumn. They're very tasty, especially the juicy huckleberries. In montane areas, watch out for bears in huckleberry patches, as bear feast on huckleberries to fatten up for the winter.

Cattails

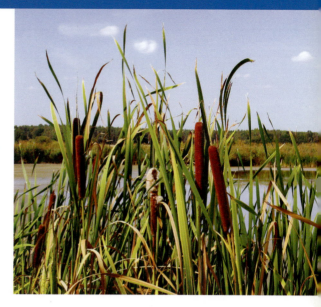

Cattail shoots and roots are edible parts of cattail plants which are referred to as "Cossack asparagus" although the tender, white shoots apparently taste more like cucumbers. The tough, fibrous cattail roots can also be dug up, dried and ground into flour or boiled down with water to separate the starch.

Cranberries

Look for the large, red, round berries of the cranberry plant along the edges of areas of muskeg or peat bogs, which should be ripe for harvesting in the autumn (especially after a frost when they taste sweeter as their sugar content increases). The berries can be eaten raw but are usually eaten as dried berries or made into a syrup as they tend to be tart. There are both high bush and low bush cranberry plants in Canada.

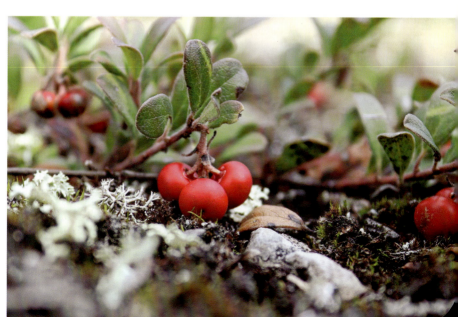

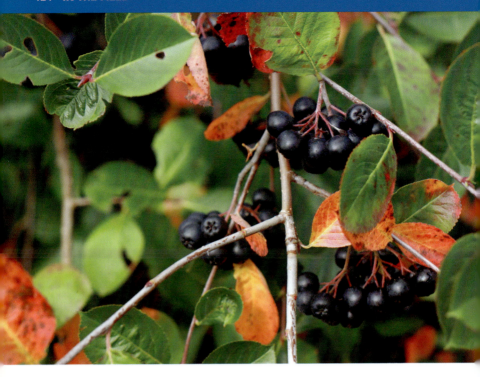

Chokecherries

The fleshy part of Canadian chokecherry berries is edible, but their seeds are poisonous. The dark purple fruit has a bitter taste. Chokecherry bushes are very common in Alberta and British Columbia and are found throughout southern Canada.

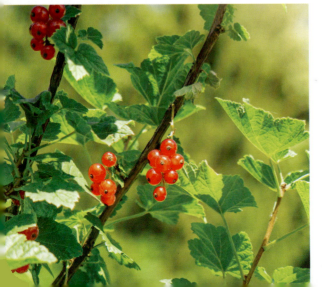

Currants

There are over a dozen species of currants in Canada that have edible fruits. The fruits range from red to bluish to black. Currants do not have spines or prickles, distinguishing them from gooseberries, which are also edible.

Morels

Morels are a distinct looking edible mushroom with a cone-shaped cap and sponge-like texture. They have a hollow inside, grow between two and four inches tall are can be dark or white in colour. They're found in old forest fire burns, fields and beside forest trails throughout Canada and are most common in the spring. Like other mushrooms, morels tend to sprout after a rain. Because raw mushrooms are hard on the human digestive system, it is best to cook (fry or grill) morels. They shouldn't be eaten raw, or you'll get sick. Morels are one of the few mushrooms that have a distinctive shape that can be easily identified and eaten safely. A true morel will be hollow inside from the tip of the cap to the bottom of the stem. **Warning: There are false morels that do not have a hollow inside that should not be eaten.**

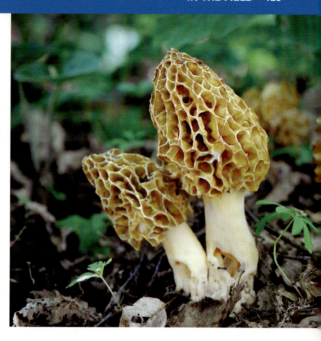

Raspberries

Wild raspberries are found in sunny areas in woods and clearings from Newfoundland to British Columbia and in the northern territories. These red berries are safe to eat and nutritious.

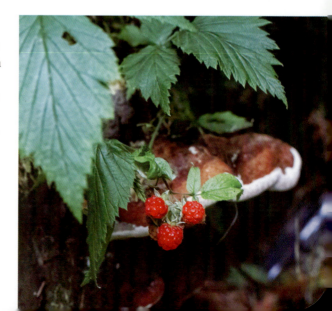

Saskatoon Berries

Saskatoon berries are very common in western Canada, especially near watercourses. The bushes attract black bears during the late summer and autumn, so keep an eye out for them.

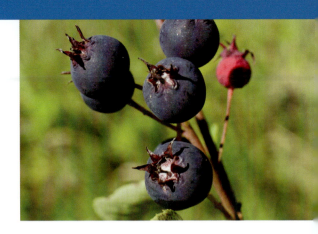

Strawberries

Wild strawberries are native to Canada, most common in the southern parts of the country and whose bright red berries are safe to eat. Wild strawberries grow in open, well-drained places in lowland to subalpine zones but are not abundant in arid parts of Canada. These plants can be found in fields and meadows, disturbed areas and open forest.

Both wild leeks and ginseng should be left alone as they are rare and endangered in Canada. Wild leeks are onion-like plants that grow in the deep woods. The leaves come up in the spring, usually before much of anything else has come up. The flowers only appear after the leaves have mostly died off. Wild ginseng should not be harvested because it is a protected species of plant.

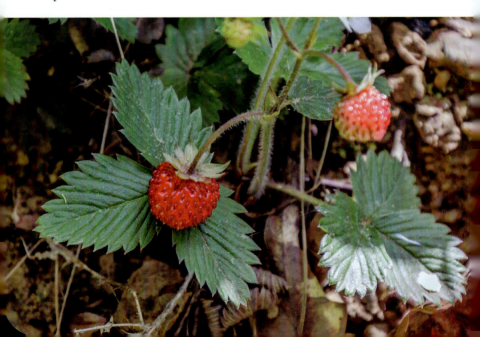

Poisonous Plants (Wild)

Some (but not all) of Canada's most dangerous wild, poisonous plants are described below:

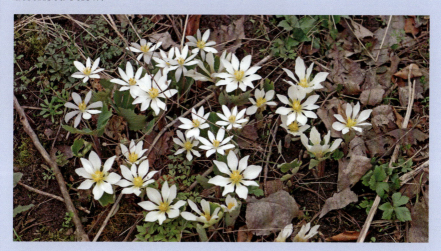

Bloodroot

Bloodroot is found from southeast Manitoba to Nova Scotia. The bloodroot flower resembles a water lily and has 8–16 white petals that surround a golden yellow centre. Bloodroot gets its name from its underground stems, also called rhizomes, that contain a red juice. The roots of bloodroot are extremely poisonous. Bloodroot's natural habitat is in or at the edge of rich, moist woods. The plant contains many alkaloids and is poisonous in large doses.

Poison Ivy and Poison Oak

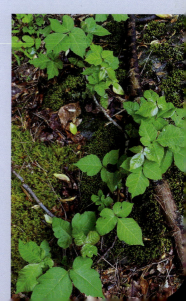

Poison ivy is an ubiquitous and famous plant that causes rashes and fever and should not be touched. Both poison ivy and poison oak plants contain an oily resin called urushiol that causes an allergic skin reaction in most people. This oil is in the leaves, stems and roots of poison ivy, poison oak and poison sumac. If you come in contact with poison ivy, you should wash your hands as soon as possible to avoid getting an ugly rash. Signs and symptoms of a poison ivy rash include redness, itching, swelling, blisters and difficulty breathing if you've inhaled smoke from burning poison ivy.

Snowberry

Snowberry, whose small berries are snow white in colour, grows from the Northwest Territories throughout most of the southern Canadian provinces. The berries are mildly poisonous but in large quantities can be toxic. Most snowberry plants are in the form of small shrubs.

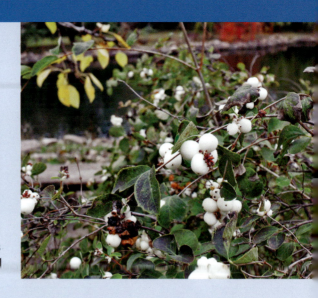

Water-Hemlocks

Water-Hemlocks (there are several different species of hemlocks) are regarded as one of Canada's most poisonous native plants and arguably one of the most dangerous plants on the North American continent. All parts of the plant contain a highly poisonous toxin called cicutoxin. Water hemlock can be found sporadically near marshes, pastures, rivers and streams. The plant can grow up to 1–2 m in height, and has a hollow, branching stem with a spotted purple pattern. It produces white flowers clustered together in the shape of an umbrella. Northern *water-hemlock* (*Cicuta virosa*) is a native perennial herb found across Canada.

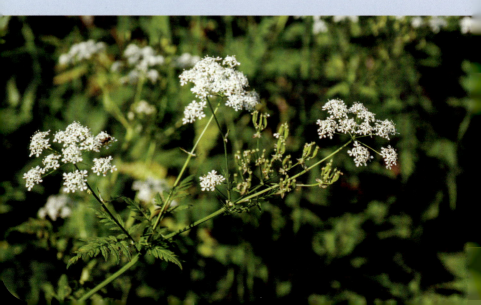

Nuts and Seeds

Wild nuts found in western Canada include the beaked hazelnut (Corylus cornuta), whitebark pine seeds (Pinus albicaulis), and garry oak acorns (Quercus garryana). Sources indicate that virtually all are known to have been used as food by Indigenous Peoples. Generally speaking, consumption of wild nuts and seeds is complicated, and references should be sourced on species that would be present in the area you intend to travel before you make a trip because they are not found everywhere. Further, they may require special treatment to make them edible because of potential toxicity issues.

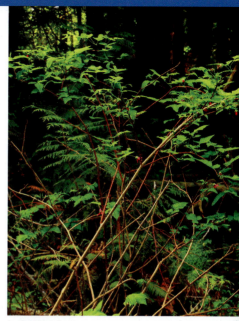
Beaked hazelnut

Bird Eggs

It's certainly possible to source bird eggs in many parts of Canada during the spring mating and nesting season, especially those of waterfowl which usually nest near waterbodies in dense grasses. Canada geese and duck nests would be the most likely sources of eggs. Hold an egg up against a light source (e.g., a flashlight) to ensure the inside contents are translucent for quality eggs where the embryo hasn't yet developed. If the whole egg is dark, there's a chick inside. It would be very difficult to find the nests of upland game birds which are generally well hidden.

Canada geese eggs

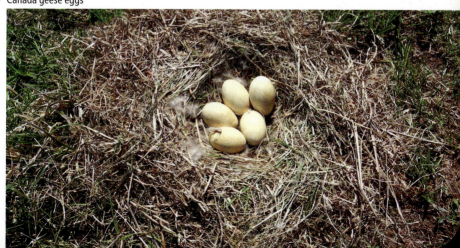

Insects

Grasshoppers and crickets are noted for being rich in protein and are found throughout most of southern Canada. Most types of grasshoppers and crickets are edible but should be cooked before they are eaten as they can carry nematodes (i.e., round worms). It's easiest to collect them in the morning when it's cold and their bodies haven't warmed up. To prepare crickets and grasshoppers, pull off their heads and the entrails and discard both. Remove the wings and legs. Dry roast the remains if you have a pan or skewer them and roast over flame if you don't.

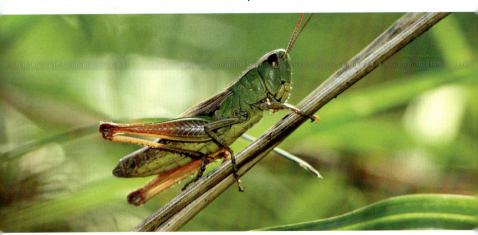

Ants are also edible. Capture as many as you can with your hands and put them into a can filled with water so that they drown while you catch more. Once you've caught a bunch of ants, boil them for about six minutes to neutralize the acid in their bodies. If you have to eat them raw, make sure they're dead first otherwise they'll bite you. Anthills are the motherlode for collecting them or look under rocks and boulders or dead, fallen trees.

If your stomach can handle it, you could also collect wood lice (commonly referred to a sow bugs in Canada) which are actually a form of crustacean and are very common in and around wooded areas in rotten, fallen trees, etc. Put them in boiling water and boil them for several minutes to kill nematodes they may be carrying (parasitic roundworms) which can infect your intestines, so be sure they're thoroughly cooked. When they're done, strain the water out and eat them.

Earthworms can also be eaten in a pinch after they've been pinched to rid them of bodily wastes and boiled to sterilize them.

Do not try to eat bees or wasps—which can sting you and might actually kill some people with allergic reactions—or caterpillars, some of which are toxic.

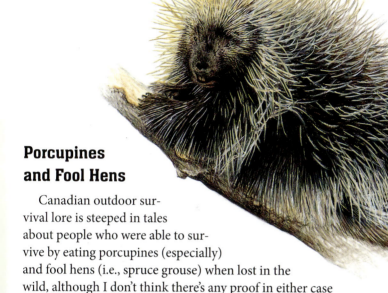

Porcupines and Fool Hens

Canadian outdoor survival lore is steeped in tales about people who were able to survive by eating porcupines (especially) and fool hens (i.e., spruce grouse) when lost in the wild, although I don't think there's any proof in either case regarding such claims. Animal traps, however, have their place in obtaining food in an emergency.

Porcupines

Porcupines are found throughout much of Canada south of the tree line, with the exception of Newfoundland and Prince Edward Island. When I was a kid, I was always told by adults not to harm porcupines because they could be killed for food if I was lost. Porcupines are not overly abundant but have a wide range in the mountains of western Canada and in the boreal forest, aspen parklands and prairies. They are large rodents that move slowly and are therefore fairly easy to kill in an emergency. The downside is that they have a huge tail full of barbed quills. When alive, they will thrash their tail against an enemy with grave consequences. Often, they curl up into a ball when threatened, turn their backs towards an enemy in self-defense or climb a nearby tree. Most animals give porcupines a wide berth and leave them alone. I've never eaten a porcupine, but I have heard that while their meat is a bit strong, it is tasty and edible. They would have to be skinned with a (pocket) knife before being butchered and cooked.

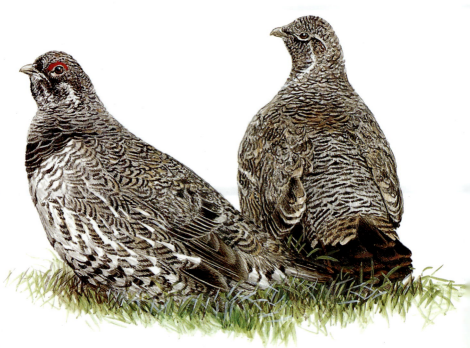

Fool Hens

Fool hens, or spruce grouse, are fairly common in the mountains and boreal forest throughout Canada. They are a dark-coloured, medium-sized grouse with a red eye patch on their head. They can be incredibly stupid (at times), making them easy to kill and eat in an emergency. They have a dark meat which can take on a turpentine flavour later on in the winter months, but are otherwise good to eat. You can kill them by throwing a stick or rock at them. To prepare a grouse for a meal, lay it on its back with its head facing away from you and put your feet on top of each wing. Next, slowly pull on each leg evenly (at the same time) to detach the bird's body from its legs, which don't have much meat on them anyway. It will free of its innards, feathers, head, etc. and will be ready to cook over a campfire. Note that it is unlawful to hunt all game birds in Canada except during an open season and only with a valid licence. Your conscience will have to be your guide if you kill a grouse out of season in an emergency. Porcupines, on the other hand, are not a protected species.

Animal Snares and Traps

An advantage of animal snares and traps is that they work 24 hours a day whereas hunting does not. Two of the most common animal snares and traps are the rabbit snare and deadfall animal trap. Set up several snares and traps to increase your chances of success.

Rabbit Snare

A rabbit snare is designed to catch snowshoe hares, which are relatively common in the boreal forest. The difference between a rabbit and a "hare" is that rabbits do not change colour in winter. The snowshoe hare is not to be confused with a "jack rabbit" or "Arctic hare", both of which are similar but larger species. Jack rabbits are distributed across the shortgrass prairies and aspen parklands, while Arctic hares are found in the barren grounds.

A rabbit snare consists of a wire attached to a tree or branch just off the ground with a loop at the end that will be pulled tight when an animal puts its head through it. Rabbit snares should be made of flexible 18–24 gauge solid wire in brass, copper or stainless steel, which will also catch red squirrels. Setting a rabbit snare is an easy, simple way to catch rabbits, and you can set one

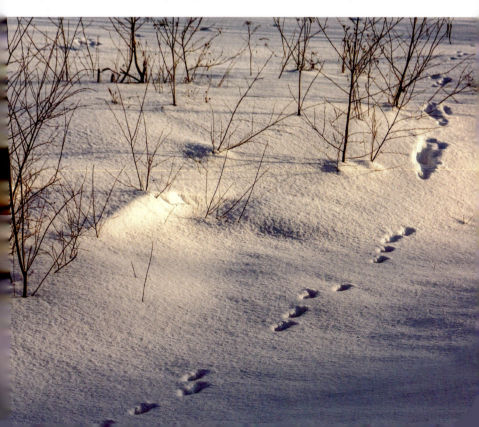

up in just a few minutes. You want your snare to be 5–6 inches off the ground. When tying the loop, remember that a rabbit needs to fit its head and ears into the trap. Most rabbits are 6–7 inches long from nose to ear tips, so the loop should be a little bit larger than the size of your fist. Start by making a small loop at the tag end, feed the wire though the loop and then fasten/anchor it to a branch or tree.

Snowshoe hares tend to travel along established forest trails in deep snow. Check for droppings—small, brown fecal pellets—to confirm their presence. To improve your odds of catching a rabbit, however, you should tramp down a trail, making it is easy for a rabbit to travel, and set your snare along the trail. Position the loop in your snare in the middle of the trail. It is also a good idea to build a "corral" using branches around the set so the rabbit doesn't go off the trail. Another trick is to place a small stick in the ground just below the loop in the snare, so the rabbit lifts its head upwards into the snare.

Deadfall Trap

A deadfall trap consists of a heavy log positioned over a bait, so when an animal takes the bait, it will trip the set and cause the log to fall down, killing the animal. One end of the log is propped up (at an angle) with a stick (branch). A cord is tied to the bottom of the stick and the bait at the other end. Another, short stick in the shape of a "Y" is pushed into the ground over the cord, so when an animal moves the bait, the stick moves and the log topples over on top of the animal.

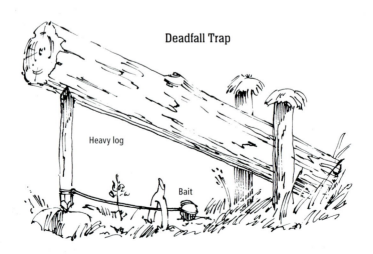

Deadfall Trap

Heavy log

Bait

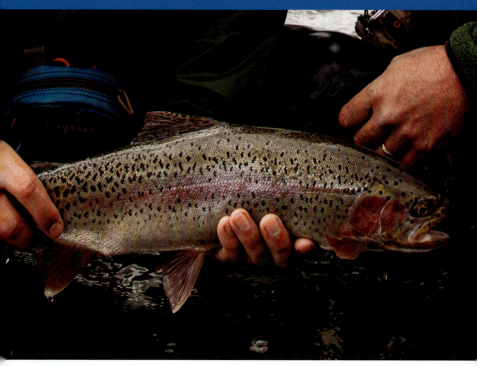

Rainbow trout

Fishing

Survival Fishing Techniques

There are a number of techniques for catching fish in a survival situation some of which, but not all, would have application in the Canadian wilderness:

- **Hand Fishing** is as primitive as fishing can get, but it usually isn't practical in Canada compared with other countries where fish behaviour is more conducive to this practice. Personally, I have captured trout by hand when they had been stranded in riverside pools, but it is almost impossible to catch them otherwise.

- **Gill nets** are used to catch fish as they try to swim though the openings of the net and become entangled in the mesh. They cannot be used legally in Canada without a licence, although Indigenous peoples can be exempted subject to various conditions across the country. They are difficult to set in a lake without a boat but could be set in streams if they were shallow enough to wade.

- **Dip nets** can be used to catch some species of fish with a dip net on their spawning grounds but rare, so a seine net would be more practical.

- *Fish spears* are useful for catching some species of fish such as bull trout on their spawning beds in small streams in the mountains of Alberta and British Columbia in the autumn, or salmon in frog water on coastal streams in British Columbia and Yukon where they rest during spawning runs.
- *Fish poisons* such as Rotenone, a fish toxicant, can be used, but it is illegal to use this toxicant in Canada without training and only then subject to taking a pesticide licence course.
- *Hand lines* are the most effective technique to catch fish. Toss a hook that's baited on the end of a line into the water to catch fish such as char and trout, in particular. They will usually hook themselves when they take the bait.
- *Gorge hooks* are baited hooks handheld until swallowed by a fish, then set by raising the fishing line. The only difference between hand lines and gorge hooks is the manner in which they are fished.
- *Striking irons* can be used to catch a large, slow-moving fish can be stunned by striking it with a rod or slender bar of metal as the fish nears the surface. It would be difficult to strike a fish in Canada using this method unless you had a boat.
- *Basket trap* used in combination with a fish weir. A container with a funnel-shaped entrance could be built as an effective fish trap, that also features a weir (e.g., rocks that would direct fish toward the entrance) to catch species that migrate, such as salmon in shallow water.

Bull trout

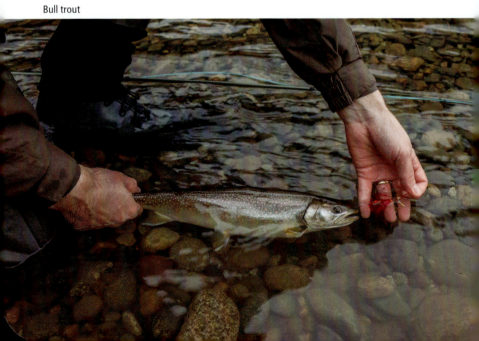

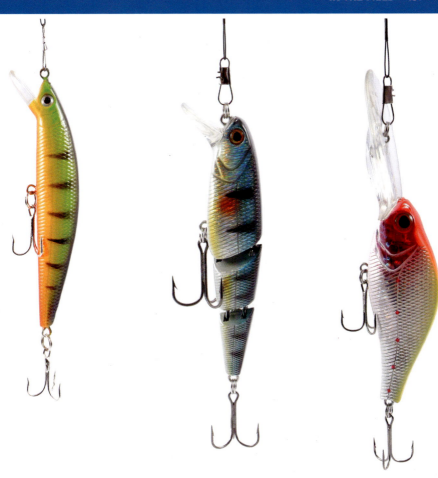

DIY Fishing Hooks

While it is possible to make DIY fishing hooks at home if you have the right material, I'm not aware of any practical techniques in the field. Survival fishing techniques are best learned in a Fishing Education Course.

Survivalist Hunting and Fishing Legalities

It is against the law to hunt or fish without a licence in Canada, so it would up the courts to decide on a course of action should a game warden find a person in violation of these laws.

Wilderness First Aid

You can't be too careful in the outdoors. One misstep might disable a person, miles from help while hiking on steep or slippery terrain. Falls are one of the most common accidents that might happen to people in Canada's outdoors, which might result in sprained ankles and fractured legs, wrists or arms. Interestingly, in the two seminal books by R. M. Patterson and George Whalley often referenced in this book, both authors make reference to various people being "laid up" from mishaps several times, often for weeks on end, which leads me to believe they had probably broken or sprained an ankle or perhaps had a tear in a meniscus in their knees.

An experience I had in March 2018 in New South Wales, Australia, typifies how injuries can occur suddenly and far from help. I was on a hunting trip for Sambar deer with a local who was an experienced hunter, familiar with the area we were hunting. I had no idea that the hunting area was going to be so rugged. As we travelled along a trail farther and farther from our trailhead, waves of kangaroos rose from their beds and scattered in front of us. The terrain became steeper and, in some cases, we had to crawl over rocky cliffs to move forward. Late in the morning I slipped on a game trail that was covered with fallen leaves. Because I was carrying a rifle with a left-handed bolt action it was shouldered on my left side so the bolt wouldn't stick in my side. The rifle was a loaner and worried me when I discovered the night before the hunt that its owner was left-handed. Normally, I would have carried a rifle with a right-handed bolt and if I fell, I would have rolled so as not to damage the rifle scope, which is expensive. This wasn't possible because the rifle was shouldered on my left side and I twisted my leg as I fell on the slippery slope. As soon as I hit the ground, I knew I was in trouble. I immediately felt a lump in my ankle that I later learned was a clinical symptom of a "spiral fracture" of the tibia. The pain was incredible, enough to make a person cry. My hunting guide, Jay Williams, and I were miles from his vehicle in an area Hollywood could have used as a set for the movie Jurassic Park. All I could do was hobble back to the trailhead. It was not fun. Later, x-rays at a local hospital in Alexandra confirmed that I had a broken leg. I was to spend the next eight weeks wearing a walking boot.

Had I not been travelling, the physician would have put my leg in a plaster cast. I'm an experienced outdoorsman, so if this sort of accident can happen to me, it can happen to just about anyone in a heartbeat.

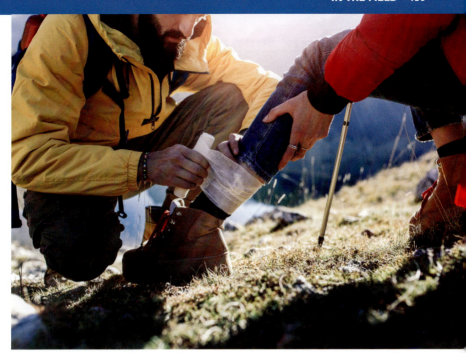

You must be properly prepared for medical emergencies (i.e., injuries and illnesses). This is why advanced training in first aid—not just basic first aid instruction—is recommended for all outdoorspeople, particularly for at-risk activities like hunting, mountain climbing and snowmobiling. All members of a party should have first aid training, because you never know who will need care. The St. John's Ambulance and Red Cross are two Canadian organizations that offer first aid courses with basic wilderness first aid training. It is incumbent on you to take these or similar courses to deal with matters of first aid that are simply too complicated to be addressed in this book.

The basic objectives of first aid are to (1) preserve life, (2) minimize the effects of injury and (3) relieve pain and suffering. Only injuries that are not life threatening (or those which might become life threatening if not treated) will be discussed here. Hunter education courses are also available locally in provinces and territories, some of which can be taken online, that also address more advanced first aid training. Courses of this nature provide a good introduction to key first aid procedures.

Ensure that members of your group have adequate health insurance, up to and including medivac services, because you may have to cover all rescue costs. Avoid solo trips in the outdoors. If you are alone and become hurt or injured, there will be no one to perform first aid or call for help.

Triage (ABCDE Rule)

Medical teams use a systematic method for managing all acutely ill patients and clinical emergencies called the ABCDE (A–E) Approach.

It is a way of systematically assessing each of a patient's vital systems—airway, breathing, circulation, disability, and exposure—to diagnose and treat injuries.

ABCDE Rule

The letters in the acronym stand for:

A-airway

B-breathing

C-circulation

D-disability

E-exposure

The objectives of the ABCDE approach are to:
- provide life-saving treatment
- break down complex clinical situations into more manageable parts
- serve as an assessment and treatment algorithm
- establish common situational awareness among all treatment providers
- buy time to establish a final diagnosis and treatment

If a person is on the ground, start by lifting their head and tilting their chin to make sure their **airway** is open. Next, look, listen and feel for signs of **breathing**. To assess their **circulation,** feel for a pulse and pinch a finger to assess capillary refill time (i.e., recirculation). Determine their level of **disability** by seeing if they're alert, respond to voices, whether they're pain responsive or unresponsive. Lastly, **exposure** by removal of clothing is the final step to assess the nature of possible injuries.

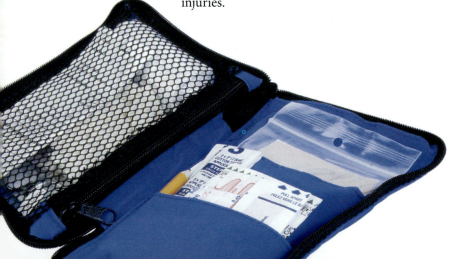

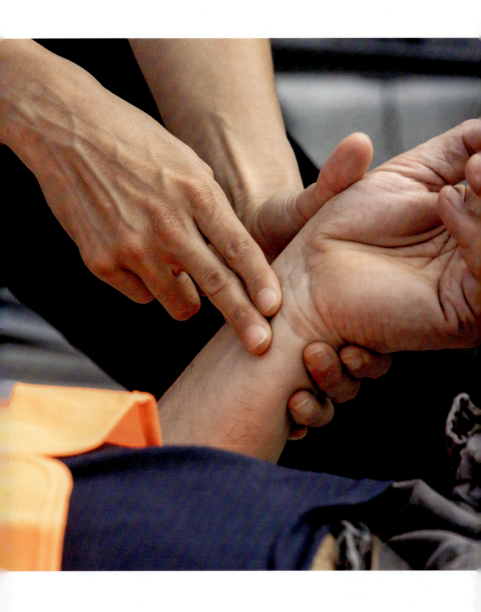

CPR

It is important to be familiar with cardiopulmonary resuscitation (CPR), which can be a lifesaving technique in many emergencies, including a heart attack or drowning, in which someone's breathing or heartbeat has stopped. For example, you must be familiar with how to administer mouth-to-mouth resuscitation and chest pressure using the arm lift method should the mouth-to-mouth method not be possible due to mouth or facial injuries. These key life-saving procedures require training to undertake properly.

CPR training is not simple; the Red Cross course involves up to **3 hours of online learning and 3 hours of in-person teaching time, and online learning may vary depending on the student.**

The basic CPR life support steps until medical help arrives or in the case of dire emergencies are as follows:

1. Call 911 or ask someone else for Emergency Medical Services assistance. (If you can't call 911, proceed to Step 2.)
2. Lay the person on their back and open their airways.
3. Check for signs of breathing. If they are not breathing, start CPR.
4. Perform 30 chest compressions.
5. Perform two rescue breaths.
6. Repeat until an ambulance or, in the case of a heart attack, an automated external defibrillator (AED) arrives.

In the case of a drowning, turn the drowning person's head to the side, allowing any water to drain from his or her mouth and nose. Next, turn the head back to the centre. Begin mouth-to-mouth resuscitation on land, if possible, or in the water if the injured person needs immediate attention.

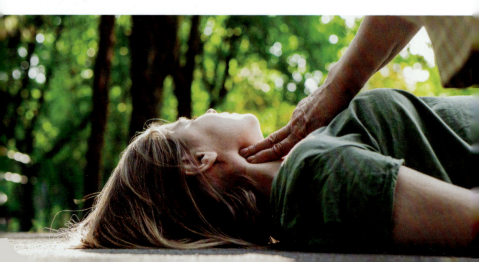

Before Giving CPR

1. Check the scene and the person. Make sure the scene is safe, then tap the person on the shoulder and shout "Are you OK?" to ensure that the person needs help.

2. Call 911 for assistance. If it's evident that the person needs help, call (or ask a bystander to call) 911, then send someone to get an AED. (If an AED is unavailable, or a there is no bystander to access it, stay with the victim, call 911 and begin administering assistance.)

3. Open the airway. With the person lying on his or her back, tilt the head back slightly to lift the chin.

4. Check for breathing. Listen carefully, for no more than 10 seconds, for sounds of breathing. (Occasional gasping sounds do not equate to breathing.) If there is no breathing begin CPR.

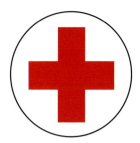

Red Cross CPR Steps

1. Push hard, push fast. Place your hands, one on top of the other, in the middle of the chest. Use your body weight to help you administer compressions that are at least 2 inches deep and delivered at a rate of at least 100 compressions per minute.

2. Deliver rescue breaths. With the person's head tilted back slightly and the chin lifted, pinch the nose shut and place your mouth over the person's mouth to make a complete seal. Blow into the person's mouth to make the chest rise. Deliver two rescue breaths, then continue compressions.
Note: If the chest does not rise with the initial rescue breath, re-tilt the head before delivering the second breath. If the chest doesn't rise with the second breath, the person may be choking. After each subsequent set of 30 chest compressions, and before attempting breaths, look for an object and, if seen, remove it.

3. Continue CPR steps. Keep performing cycles of chest compressions and breathing until the person exhibits signs of life, such as breathing, an AED becomes available, or EMS or a trained medical responder arrives on scene.
Note: End the cycles if the scene becomes unsafe or you cannot continue performing CPR due to exhaustion.

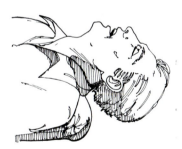

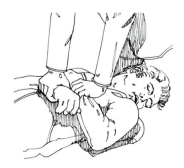

Frostbite: Signs, Treatment and Prevention

Frostbite

Canada is one of the coldest countries in the world, which is why both frostbite and hypothermia must always be an issue of concern regarding outdoor survival.

According to the Mayo Clinic, "frostbite is an injury caused by freezing of the skin and underlying tissues. First your skin becomes very cold and red, then numb, hard and pale." Often a person may not realize they have frostbite, so it's always a good idea to travel in a group and to watch out for fellow travelers. Frostbite is most common on the fingers, toes, nose, ears, cheeks and chin. Exposed skin in cold, windy weather is most vulnerable to frostbite. Wear a jacket with a fur-lined hood to help prevent frostbite on your face. Research reported in *Men's Journal* found that lined (e.g., wolf, wolverine, fox) hoods effectively reduced exposure to the cold by preventing frost from building up around the face.

> **Often a person may not realize they have frostbite, so it's always a good idea to travel in a group and to watch out for fellow travelers.**

If medical help is not available take appropriate self-care measures, such as:

- Protecting the affected area from further cold and warming it to body temperature
- Not walking on frostbitten feet
- Reducing pain with ibuprofen (Advil, Motrin IB, others)

Frostbite is exacerbated by wind when temperatures are below 0°C. While being "cold" is a relative term, science dictates that the danger of frostbite increases with wind speed. Research indicates that once the wind chill makes the temperature feel like −28°C or colder, exposed skin can freeze in under 30 minutes. When it drops to −40°C, frostbite can occur in less than 10 minutes. At temperatures below 0°C, a person's blood vessels start to constrict and shunt blood from their extremities to preserve core body temperature. When that happens fingers, toes and a person's face, in particular, can quickly freeze. Lined mittens, rather than finger gloves, keep in heat the best, so they're better at preventing your fingers from freezing. There are many cases where outdoorspeople have lost fingers and toes due to frostbite, so it shouldn't be taken lightly.

The Sourtoe Cocktail:

There's a slogan in the Downtown Hotel in Dawson City, Yukon: "You can drink it fast; you can drink it slow, but your lips must touch the toe…" in reference to the Sourtoe Cocktail Club ritual. Established in 1973 by the late Captain Dick Stevenson, the Sourtoe Cocktail Club induction ceremony has become a Dawson City tradition and is exactly what is sounds like: an actual human toe, amputated due to frostbite that has been dehydrated and preserved in salt, is used to garnish a drink of your choice. As the saying goes, your lips must touch the toe as you down your drink. I'm an official member of the Sourtoe Cocktail Club, having been inducted by Captain Stevenson, which I imbibed with some Yukon Jack whiskey.

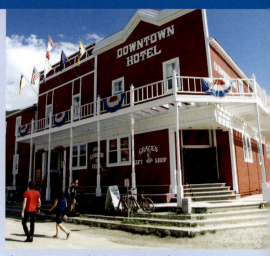

The Downtown Hotel in Dawson City, Yukon

Symptoms of Frostbite

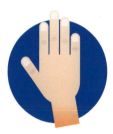

1st degree: skin whitening, reduced sensitivity

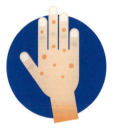

2nd degree: emergence of blisters

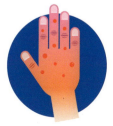

3rd degree: death of skin and subcutaneous tissues

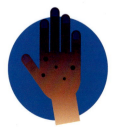

4th degree: death of skin, soft tissues and bones

Hypothermia: Signs, Treatment and Prevention

Hypothermia is a medical emergency that occurs when your body loses heat faster than it can produce heat, causing a dangerously low body temperature. Normal body temperature is around 98.6°F (37°C). Hypothermia occurs as your body temperature falls below 95°F (35° C). When your body temperature drops, your heart, nervous system and other organs can't work normally. Left untreated, hypothermia can lead to complete failure of your heart and respiratory system and eventually death. Hypothermia is often caused by exposure to cold weather or immersion in cold water.

Primary treatments for hypothermia are methods to warm the body back to a normal temperature. The most obvious symptom of hypothermia is shivering, which is the body's automatic defense against cold temperatures and an attempt to warm itself. As a person's extremities get cold, the body also reacts by trying to warm the inside of the torso where vital organs are located. Other symptoms include slurred speech, mumbling, slow shallow breathing, a weak pulse, lack of coordination, drowsiness, a loss of consciousness and often bright red skin, with cold skin in infants. A person with hypothermia sometimes isn't aware of his or her condition because the symptoms often begin gradually. It has been my observation that it often follows extreme exertion in cold weather and triggers extreme shivering. It is essential that they be warmed up to prevent a medical emergency.

Frostbite may be a precursor of *hypothermia,* which occurs when a person's body loses heat faster than it can produce heat and their body temperature falls below 35°C, or when their inner body temperature drops more than two degrees Celsius. When a person is said to have died from "exposure," often the actual cause of death was hypothermia. It can also be caused by ongoing exposure to

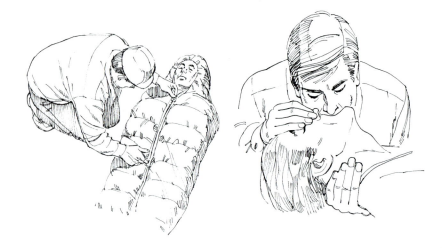

indoor temperatures below 10°C. It is accelerated by wet or damp clothing, wind, exhaustion and sudden contact with cold water, or immersion. If let uncorrected, it can be deadly. Signs and symptoms of hypothermia include: shivering, slurred speech or mumbling, and slow, shallow breathing. Hypothermia impairs a person's ability to think and act rationally. As a person's body temperature decreases, vital internal organs (brain, liver, heart) lose their ability to function. Victims first experience uncontrollable shivering, followed by confusion, memory loss, unconsciousness and possibly death.

Even mild hypothermia requires treatment. A victim of hypothermia may deny they are in trouble, so the best advice is to believe what you see, not what the victim might say.

Take the following steps to treat a person with hypothermia:

1. Move the victim to warm shelter as soon as possible. If a shelter isn't readily available, build a fire.
2. Remove the victim's clothes if they are wet.
3. Apply heat to the victim's head, neck, chest and groin with warm moist towels, hot water bottles or heated blankets. Replace these items as they cool off with warm packs.
4. If a sleeping bag is available, put the victim in the bag, remove your clothing and lay close to the person, inside the bag if possible, to transfer your body heat to theirs.
5. As the person recovers, give them something warm to drink to help raise their core body temperature. Don't give them alcohol, which will lower their core body temperature.

Be prepared: check the weather forecast before you go, wear clothing that will keep you dry and warm, check your partner(s) for symptoms regularly and have a survival kit in your jacket pocket in case of an emergency.

C.O.L.D.

Use the C.O.L.D. acronym for judging your clothing against the elements:

C-clean

O-(avoid) overheating

L-loose and in layers

D-dry

Dirty garments will not keep you warm, and you don't want to wear too many clothes or you might get overheated, which is one of the key reasons for wearing loose clothing and in layers.

Dehydration: Signs and Treatment

It is important to stay hydrated while outdoors. Otherwise you can develop a headache, get dizzy and lose your balance. Seniors in particular need to be cognizant of this requirement, because they often don't drink enough water in the first place. Dehydration could cause you to make missteps or fall and hurt yourself. Sip water during the day to stay hydrated—more so on hot days when you're expending a lot of energy. The amount of water you'll need varies according to the length and difficulty of the trial and weather conditions.

Heatstroke and Heat Exhaustion: Signs, Treatment and Prevention

Back in the day, heatstroke was commonly referred to as "sunstroke," which is the same thing. I had mild cases of sunstroke a couple of times as a youngster and neither was any fun.

Heatstroke is caused by your body overheating, usually as a result of prolonged exposure to or physical exertion in high temperatures. In young people just being outside in the heat of summer can cause mild forms of heatstroke, which is one good reason to always wear a hat to shield your head from the sun. People of any age, however, can experience heatstroke. Heatstroke can occur if your body temperature rises to 104°F (40°C) or higher, which is most common in the summer. Heatstroke should be treated seriously and requires emergency treatment. Untreated heatstroke can quickly damage a person's brain, heart, kidneys and muscles. The damage worsens the longer treatment is delayed, increasing your risk of serious complications or death. Symptoms include not only a high body temperature but cognitive failure, nausea and vomiting, flushed skin, rapid breathing, a racing heart rate and often a bad headache. People who are experiencing heat stroke should get medical aid as soon as possible. You should take immediate action to cool the overheated person while waiting for emergency treatment.

> **Heatstroke should be treated seriously and requires emergency treatment. Untreated heatstroke can quickly damage a person's brain, heart, kidneys and muscles.**

The Mayo Clinic recommends the following course of action:
- Get the person into shade or indoors.
- Remove excess clothing.

Cool the person with whatever means available—in a cool tub of water or a cool shower, spray with a garden hose, sponge with cool water, fan while misting with cool water, or place ice packs or cold, wet towels on the person's head, neck, armpits and groin.

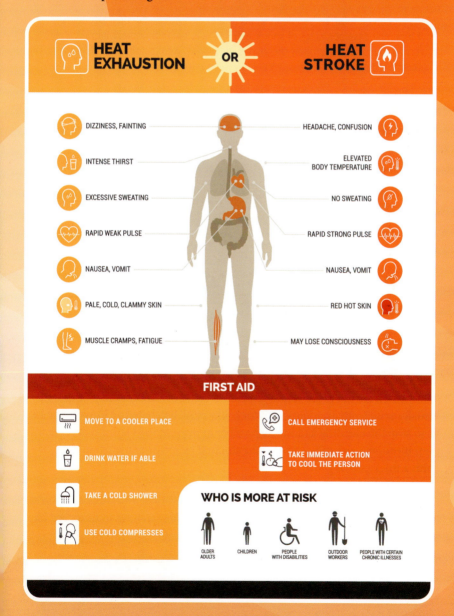

Shock: Signs and Treatment

A victim of any kind of accident or medical emergency will often experience "shock" in addition to their injuries. Shock can happen immediately or several hours after an accident. A person in shock will be pale, perspiring and feel faint. Their pulse will be rapid and weak, and their skin will feel cold and damp.

> Shock can be fatal, so people in shock require immediate medical attention. If a person develops signs of shock, call 911 and begin treatment immediately. (If you can't call 911, follow the guidelines below.) Adults and older children experiencing shock will usually have several symptoms, including:
>
> · Passing out (losing consciousness)Feeling dizzy or light-headed.
>
> · Feeling weak or having trouble standing.
>
> · Not feeling alert or able to think clearly. They may be confused, restless, fearful or unable to respond to questions.

It is best to keep a victim experiencing shock laying down with their head raised slightly if they have an injury to the head or neck. A person in shock loses heat rapidly, so it is important to keep them warm by covering them with a blanket or coat and placing a blanket underneath them if the ground is cold.

Wounds: Treatment and Preventing Infection

Bleeding

Proper first aid training is also required to attend to serious bleeding from cuts, which are likely the outdoorsperson's most common injury. Such cuts usually arise from accidents with tools like axes, hatchets and knives. The key is to stop the bleeding as soon as possible to prevent the victim from bleeding out. Bleeding from most cuts can be stopped by pressing firmly on the cut with a thick pad of gauze or cloth.

In serious cases, it may be necessary to use a tourniquet, but only if a victim's life is endangered. Use common sense regarding application of a tourniquet. If a person is losing a lot of blood, you're going to have to tie a cord like a shoelace above the cut to stop the bleeding or before the loss of blood becomes fatal. Once the bleeding stops—if it does—the tourniquet can be removed. Note that tissue damage can occur if the tourniquet is applied too long. This is a judgement call. Medical tourniquets are available for emergency use and would be a good investment for a first aid kit.

The best thing to do is take a course on the proper procedure to deal with bleeding from cuts, because even the basics are complicated.

Cuts and Infections

Cuts are likely the most common injuries that outdoorspeople suffer from. It is very important to treat cuts and bruises with a disinfectant to prevent infections, which can be deadly if they turn septic.

If a patient becomes "septic," they will likely have low blood pressure leading to poor circulation and lack of blood perfusion of vital tissues and organs. They will experience chills or rigors (i.e., usually characterized with shivering at the onset of high fever and chills). This is a form of "blood poisoning" that represents a serious and sometimes fatal infection. Septicemia occurs when a bacterial infection elsewhere in the body, such as the lungs or skin, enters the bloodstream. This is dangerous because the bacteria and their toxins can be carried through the bloodstream to your entire body. Septicemia can quickly become life-threatening. Sepsis can kill a person within 12 hours. Medical attention is required for cuts that become infected, and people who show signs of sepsis require urgent medical attention (see Emergency Communications in Part 3) and need to be hospitalized. Sepsis is treated with antibiotics, often administered over a period of several days. Patients may also require oxygen and intravenous fluids to maintain blood flow to circulate oxygenated blood.

There are two kinds of disinfectants mentioned in the first aid kits (see First Aid Kit on page 46). The first, Benzalkonium chloride wipes, also known as towelettes, are used as a skin disinfectant. They are ideal for cleansing a wound and are effective against bacteria, viruses, fungi and protozoa. Second, Merthiolate swabs are used to prevent skin infections and clean wounds. This first aid product contains the active ingredient Benzalkonium and effectively disinfects the affected area. It is ideal for treating minor scrapes, cuts and burns.

Broken Bones and Sprains

Next to cuts, sprains are the most commonly reported injury suffered by outdoorspeople. This is an important section because it should be possible for outdoorspeople to administer self-treatment for these all-too-common backcountry injuries. Further, by properly dealing with broken bones and ankle sprains, you can buy some time while waiting for professional medical help to arrive.

A sprain is a stretching or tearing of ligaments, which are tough bands of fibrous tissue that connect two bones together in a person's joints. The most common location for a sprain is in the ankle. Initial treatment includes rest, icing the sprained area and compression to reduce inflammation and swelling.

A fracture is a broken bone. There are two kinds of fractures: simple and compound. A simple or closed fracture is characterized by a broken bone under the surface of the skin. A compound or open fracture occurs when the broken bone cuts through the skin and makes an open wound. When this happens, you should not try to push the bone back inside and instead control bleeding by applying direct pressure before getting medical attention. Use a splint or sling to support an ankle, arm or wrist with a fracture until the victim can get medical attention.

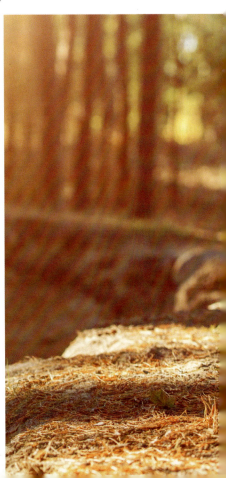

If you fall and sprain your ankle or fracture your leg, you will experience a sharp pain (at the point of fracture) and swelling almost immediately, which will get worse until treated. You will require medical treatment, including an x-ray, to determine the nature of the injury. In the case of a severe sprain or fracture, it will be very painful to walk without crutches. In fact, you may cause more harm if you try walking on a fractured leg or sprained ankle. To help reduce swelling, you need to elevate the appendage and apply ice packs. Compression bandages will also provide important relief and reduce swelling. Most spiral fractures involve the long bones of the legs, such as the femur, tibia and fibula. The injury can also involve the long bones of the arms, including the humerus, ulna and radius. Spiral fractures are common when a person puts out an arm or quickly repositions their leg to try and catch themselves while falling. If you are able to, try to roll with an anticipated fall instead and you may be able to prevent a sprain or spiral fracture.

A dislocation is the displacement of the end of a bone from its joint. Dislocations have the same symptoms as fractures and should be treated as if they were broken bones. Only a doctor or emergency first responder is qualified to "set" a broken bone. If you suspect a person has a back injury, take great care to immobilize them on a stretcher while taking the victim to a hospital.

In dire cases, you may have to leave a person in the backcountry to find help if the injured person unable to walk. This is a judgement call.

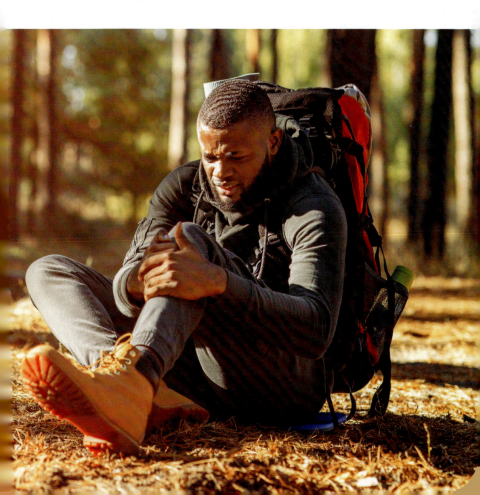

Head Injuries and Concussions: Signs and Treatment

If a person falls and injures their head, it's possible that they will suffer a concussion. Sources indicate that most people with minor head injuries recover without any problems. Keep in mind, however, that some symptoms (headaches, dizziness, difficulty concentrating) may only improve slowly over 6 to 12 weeks. Recovery will probably be slower in people whose injuries resulted in long periods of unconsciousness or amnesia. If a person loses consciousness after a fall tilt their head back, ensure their airway is clear and look/feel for signs of breathing. In the old days a person was said to be "knocked out cold" under these circumstances. Give chest compressions if they're not breathing: push firmly downwards in the middle of the chest and then release.

If a person loses consciousness after a fall tilt their head back, ensure their airway is clear and look/feel for signs of breathing.

It is not that uncommon for a person to faint for unknown reasons. If possible, lift the person's legs above heart level to aid blood flow to the brain. Feeling lightheaded and weak and having the sensation of spinning are warning signs of fainting. If you notice any of these signs, sit and put your head between your knees to help get blood to your brain. You could also lie down to avoid injury due to falling. Don't stand up until you feel better.

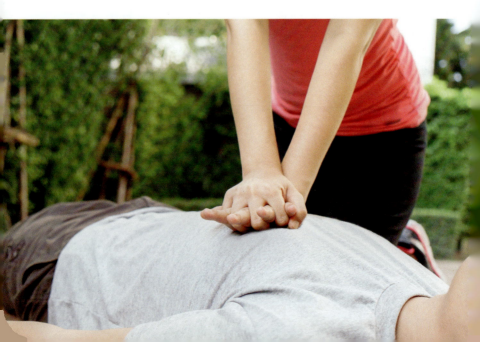

Eye Injuries

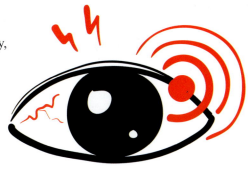

In the event of an eye injury, apply a cold compress, but don't put pressure on the eye. Take over-the-counter acetaminophen (Tylenol) or ibuprofen (Advil, Motrin) for pain. If there is bruising, bleeding, change in vision, or it hurts when your eye moves, see a doctor as soon as possible.

Treat a scratched eye using the following directions:

- Rinse your eye with saline solution or clean water
- Blink your eye
- Pull your upper eyelid over your lower eyelid
- Wear sunglasses
- Do not rub your eye. Don't touch your eye with anything. Do not wear contact lenses. Don't use redness-relieving eye drops.

Sun and Snow Blindness

Sun or Snow blindness is a temporary loss of vision due to damage to the cornea caused by exposure to the sun's ultraviolet (UV) rays. ef A person who has snow blindness will feel disoriented, having lost their sense of direction. Snow blindness usually subsides if a person rests their eyes and stays indoors.

Wearing sunglasses or tinted goggles help to prevent snow blindness. Inuit used snow goggles, designed to reduce the amount of sunlight reflecting off the snow, to ward off snow blindness. Eyesafe™ advises that dangerously high UV exposure is a higher risk during the winter because UV rays reflect off the snow and icy surfaces, and "at higher elevations, such as on ski hills, the air is thinner and UV radiation is higher. Even in overcast conditions the UV light can still penetrate cloud cover and affect your eyes. In addition to simple discomfort, overexposure can cause photokeratitis or snow blindness."

Snake Bites

First aid for snake bites:

1. Remain calm. Even if it was a venomous snake, there is a chance that no venom or poison has even been injected into the bite.
2. Call 911. Rest and wait for instructions. You will probably be instructed to go to the nearest hospital. Remain calm and move as little as possible. This will slow the spread of venom.
3. Wash the bite area with soap and water if possible.
4. Remove any jewelry or anything tight from the bitten limb.
5. Immobilize the limb.
6. Check your immunization status afterwards and obtain a tetanus shot if needed.
7. If you think you or someone you know has been bitten by a rattlesnake, go to hospital by ambulance.

What you should NOT do:

1. Do not apply a tourniquet or anything tight on a limb subject to a snake bite.
2. Do not apply ice.
3. Do not cut or suck on the bite area.
4. Do not try to catch or kill the snake.
5. Do not take any pain medicine containing aspirin or ibuprofen.

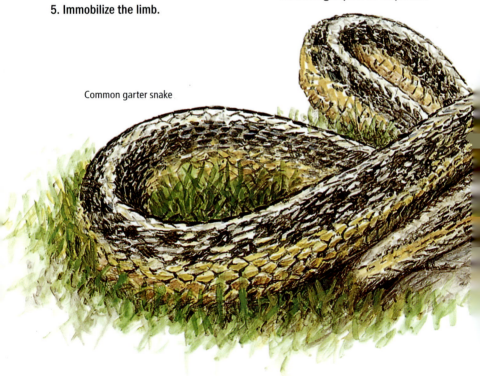

Common garter snake

Alberta Environment & Parks provides the following precautions regarding bites from snakes, because it is not just rattlesnakes that are of concern:

1. Unless you are trying to intentionally provoke, harm or capture a snake, it is very unlikely you will be bitten [by a snake].

2. In the rare event that you are bitten, the resulting wound will most likely be superficial, except in the case of the prairie rattlesnake. Bites from prairie rattlesnakes have never resulted in a fatality in Alberta, but they can be very painful and will require medical attention.

3. Snake bites, as with bites from other animals, can lead to infection. If you are bitten by a snake, even if it is not poisonous, seek medical attention to ensure that it is properly cleaned.

Insect bites

First aid recommendations for insect bites and stings:

1. Carefully remove the insect stinger or tick if still in the skin.

2. Wash the affected area with soap and water.

3. Apply a cold compress (such as a flannel or cloth cooled with cold water) or an ice pack to any swelling for at least 10 minutes.

4. Take an antihistamine (Benadryl, others) to reduce itching.

Northern River Wolf Spider

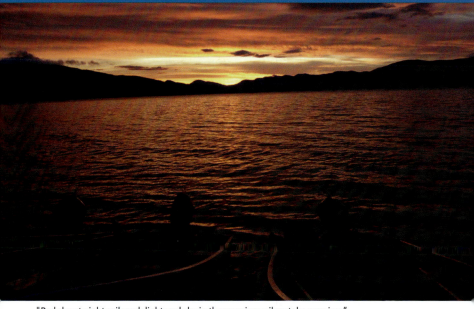

"Red sky at night sailors delight; red sky in the morning sailors take warning."

Environmental Hazards

Inclement Weather

When you're out and about in Canada's outdoors, make it a practice to take notice of the natural world around you. Nature often predicts atmospheric changes.

If you familiarize yourself with the behaviour of birds, you can watch for increased activity and changes in their feeding patterns to alert you to an incoming change in weather. Birds can signal a change in weather, often for the worst, especially summer rain and winter snowstorms. You might be surprised at how reliably bird behaviour can be used to forecast weather, which tends to come in from certain directions in different parts of Canada. There is a saying that when it's raining on the coast of British Columbia, the wind will be blowing in southern Alberta.

Canadian songbirds, as well as gulls, pigeons, crows and magpies detect changes in barometric pressure, several hours ahead of when a storm might arrive. They will feed most actively, and generally all at the same time, prior to a storm that they sense is on the horizon with uncanny accuracy.

Most songbirds feed on insects while in flight, and birds, such as swallows, tend to fly at the same height as insects because that's where their supper is! The height at which insects fly is affected by barometric pressure, which explains the link between bird feeding patterns and changes in weather. Low barometric pressure is associated with rain, so, when the barometric pressure drops, humidity goes up and air temperatures drops, causing insects to fly lower to the ground and birds to follow suit.

In contrast, high barometric pressure is associated with sunny skies and warm temperatures. High pressure systems create stable weather conditions, usually clear, fine days. When there is an absence of clouds in the sky, the prevailing weather is conducive to the buildup of warm, uplifting "thermals" that carry insects higher into the atmosphere. In response to this balmy weather, birds will fly high into the sky to catch the insects.

In the mountains of western Canada, the skies are typically clear in the morning with clouds developing in the afternoon after the ground heats up and carries moisture into the atmosphere. This leads to a risk of thundershowers later in the day, which is why you should always pack a raincoat for day hikes.

Storms can arise suddenly and swamp boats, flood campsites and drench hikers and campers, plus they are often associated with lightning strikes, which can be fatal.

There is scientific validity to the old adage, *"Red sky at night sailors delight; red sky in the morning sailors take warning."* This saying is rooted in biblical history and carries over to a converse proverb, *"Red sky at night, shepherds' delight. Red sky in the morning, shepherds' warning."*

A red sky before nightfall is normally a sign that a high-pressure system is settling in, which is generally characterized by stable weather and clear skies over the next few days. A red sky in the morning indicates bad weather is imminent and can be an indication there is rain on the way.

Canadian songbirds, as well as gulls, pigeons, crows and magpies detect changes in barometric pressure, several hours ahead of when a storm might arrive.

There are other sayings such as: *"When the dew is on the grass, Rain will never come to pass. When grass is dry at morning light, Look for rain before the night."* Usually, dew will form on a clear and calm night when temperatures chill down to the dew point; however, if no dew forms, it is probably because there was wind and warm temperatures overnight, and rain may be on the way.

Keep your eye open for dust devils during the summer, which can be a sign that the wind direction is going to change.

Landslides and Avalanches

Avalanches

According to the Government of Canada, thousands of avalanches occur in Canada each year. Avalanches happen in all parts of Canada, but are more frequent in the mountains of British Columbia, Yukon and Alberta. They can be triggered by wind, rain, warming temperatures, snow and earthquakes. They can also be triggered by skiers, snowmobiles, hikers and vibrations from machinery or construction activities.

If your trip involves skiing, climbing or snowmobiling in mountainous areas during the winter, you need to know how to identify whether you're in avalanche country, how to minimize your risk in these areas and how to conduct a rescue should an avalanche occur. The best way to learn these skills is to take an avalanche training course.

Avalanches are most common during the winter and late spring, from December to April in Canada, but they do occur year-round. An avalanche arises from a surface bed of snow (a weaker layer that can collapse) and an overlaying heavy snow slab. The highest risk period is during and immediately after a snowstorm, which puts additional weight on a cornice on precipitous mountain slopes. Avalanche slopes are steep and are often devoid of mature trees in Canada's high country. A hallmark of an avalanche slope is broken trees, often with their trunks sheared off near the ground.

In western Canada, an average of 14 people die in avalanches annually—about 80 percent of the fatalities are in British Columbia, while the rest in Alberta and Yukon. In 90 percent of avalanche accidents worldwide, the victim or someone in the victim's party causes the snow slide. Sources indicate that most deaths occurred while participating in recreational backcountry activities; 85.7 percent

> **If your trip involves skiing, climbing or snowmobiling in mountainous areas during the winter, you need to know how to identify whether you're in avalanche country, how to minimize your risk in these areas and how to conduct a rescue should an avalanche occur.**

of deaths were due to asphyxiation, 8.9 percent were due to a combination of asphyxiation and trauma and 5.4 percent were due to trauma alone (head injuries were frequent in those killed solely by trauma). The natural instinct for anyone buried by an avalanche is to panic, but if you can keep your head, you can stay alive for a while. In most cases, victims have a 15-minute window in which they can carve out an area to breathe under the snow.

It's not just your average outdoorsmen that die in avalanches. Even seasoned backcountry users have been killed. In the spring of 2019, three world-class climbers disappeared in April as they tried to descend Howse Peak in the Rocky Mountains on the continental divide between Alberta and British Columbia (*Ice climbers urged to wear avalanche safety gear, Edmonton Journal, December 23, 2019 by Colette Derworiz*). The report says that the rescue was challenging because the missing climbers were not wearing avalanche beacons. Parks Canada authorities maintain that anyone in avalanche terrain should have a safety beacon, a probe and a shovel. While it's true that climbers who get hit by an avalanche will likely get killed, there is always a chance that you can dig people out of an avalanche. However, not wearing a beacon can further endanger the lives of rescuers searching for you. It is very dangerous to attempt to recover bodies buried in an avalanche—it often takes a search dog to find the bodies—and wearing a beacon or even a RECCO strip on a headlamp can make it much more likely that you will be found.

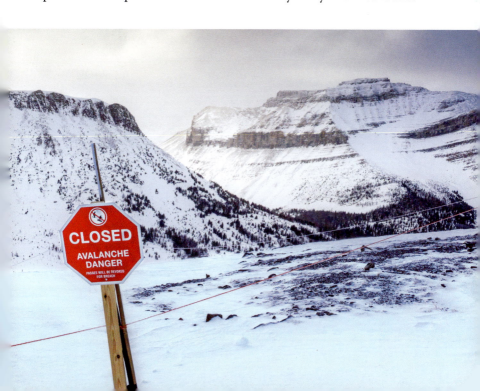

RECCO Avalanche System: The RECCO® Rescue System is a two-part system. Manufactures attach a small Band-Aid-sized reflector (sometimes called a "chip") into clothing, boots, helmets, Ortovox avalanche transceivers, etc. The reflector is a passive device and does not require batteries or any user attention. A special detector, which is used by professional rescuers, transmits a signal that is reflected back to the detector.

The Canadian Avalanche Association report on "Guidelines for Snow Avalanche Risk Determination and Mapping in Canada" outlines technical details related to avalanche hazards for commercial activities. According to the report, "Snow avalanches are the most common mountain slope hazard that threatens people, facilities and the environment in Canada." The report describes three key types of snow avalanche mapping applications in Canada:

1. Locator maps that identify potential avalanche terrain.
2. Avalanche atlas maps that provide illustrations of potential avalanche terrain for a series of locations in an avalanche area.
3. Risk maps that are used in numerous capacities including land-use planning for fixed facilities (occupied and unoccupied buildings or structures), linear risk mapping for highways, roads or railways, and maps for forestry applications.

A spring snow avalanche on a ridge in the Rocky Mountains

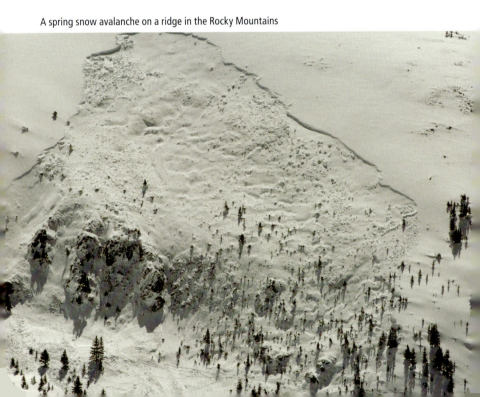

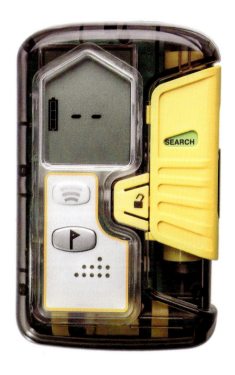

Mountain climbers, skiers and snowmobile users in avalanche country should always be equipped with an avalanche beacon, also called an avalanche transceiver.

The foregoing report is intended to understand how to minimize the avalanche risk associated with commercial activities.

Mountain climbers, skiers and snowmobile users in avalanche country should always be equipped with an avalanche beacon, also called an avalanche transceiver. These are devices that emit a pulsed radio signal and another avalanche beacon can receive this signal. They should be worn inside your clothing. All members in a team should check the battery strength of their beacon before heading out and always carry extra batteries. Remember, battery strength declines in cold weather, which is why it's best to wear a beacon against your body if possible, to capture some body heat. Cell phones and GoPro (camera) devices can disrupt signals and should be at least 12 inches away from a beacon. Make certain you and members of your team all know how beacons operate before you head out into the field. In addition to the operation of beacons, avalanche rescue authorities also recommend that users also be familiar with probing, shoveling, site control, leadership, first aid and evacuation.

Floods (Flash floods, Spring floods)

Flash floods are not uncommon anywhere in Canada, especially in the Rocky Mountains, Coastal Mountain Range and other mountain ranges where deluges often happen. Further, if heavy rains fall when the snowpack hasn't melted, flash floods can be even worse than just those arising from thunderstorms and heavy rain events during the summer. Be cautious when on rivers and streams, because flows can rise several feet in a matter of hours, making them treacherous, impossible to wade and a dangerous place to set up camp.

Fording Streams and Rivers

It can be hazardous to ford streams and rivers at any time. While the spring and summer seasons have their unique challenges, it gets even tougher in the autumn and winter when the days are short, the sun is low on the horizon (especially in the mountains) and light intensity is relatively poor.

There are some streams which are notoriously hazardous to ford year-round. For example, in the Elk River drainage in British Columbia's East Kootenay region, both Michel Creek and Lodgepole Creek have a reputation for being like skating rinks during the summer and autumn due to an infestation of algae, which blankets the substrate, and many of the streams in the Coastal Mountain Range are also treacherous because they have substrates like ball-bearings, which move under your feet as you wade through the shifting channels. Others streams, such as Goat Creek near Creston, BC, have lots of large, slippery coble in their substrate; the cobble is basically an ankle breaker in the waiting. In Labrador and in the Northern Peninsula in Newfoundland, many rivers have a substrate of large cobble, which is extremely slippery, and it's often difficult to see the stream bottom because of the tea-coloured water. Consequently, when you're fording and wading these kinds of streams, you run the risk of tripping on the substrate and falling forward (face down) or slipping and falling (most likely) backwards, or sideways. Either way, you could be in for a dunking. On some rivers, such as the Tree River in Nunavut, a fall

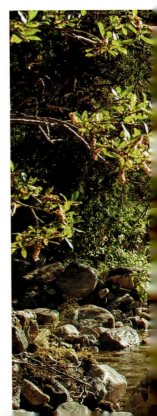

could be fatal because of its fast current. You also run the risk of spraining an ankle or breaking your leg or toes a long way from the nearest road and medical assistance.

You may need chest waders to get across some streams. You must cinch the wading belt securely around your waist at all times. If you don't properly fasten the wading belt and you fall into the water, the waders will fill with water and balloon out, which will make it very difficult for you to escape a current, and you could drown. The extra weight from the water will also make it difficult to lift yourself out of the water.

The value of a wading staff to keep your balance should not be underestimated. Wading staffs are a tremendous aid while fording streams. There are many lightweight, break-down staffs on the market that fit in holsters and can be fastened to a wading belt. In a pinch you could also use

It can be hazardous to ford streams and rivers at any time.

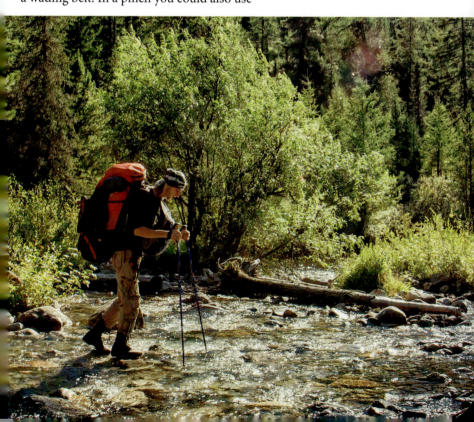

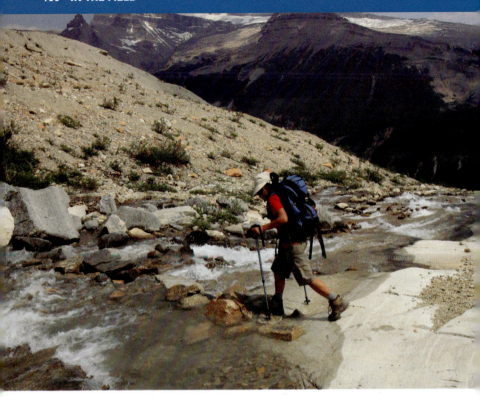

a trekking pole when fording a stream, but these tend to slip when wet and are not as safe or reliable as a commercial wading staff. A wading staff is like an extra appendage and is a great aid to maintain your balance and footing and to test the substrate before each and every step as you ford a stream. I wouldn't leave home without a wading staff, which can also be used as a substitute "trekking pole" while hiking to and from a stream.

Polarized sunglasses prevent bright sunlight and high-energy visible light from damaging or discomforting your eyes. However, they allow you to see the stream bottom because they eliminate the glare off water. I always wear polarized sunglasses when on the water during the day to protect my vision and as an aid when fording streams. If polarized glasses have a downside, it is that they darken the sky, so it can be harder to see on cloudy or foggy days or when light intensity is relatively low, which is common in autumn. On these occasions, you can wear amber sunglasses instead.

Keep your legs apart when fording a stream. Watch your step and take one step at a time. Then brace yourself before you take the next step. Once your foot is secure, move forward again. Cross streams facing upstream and move sideways so your three points of support (i.e., your feet and wading staff) form a triangle. Move crab-like to spread your weight evenly over your hips, your body's centre of gravity. If the current is swift, choose a path that takes you diagonally across and downstream so that you won't have to fight the full force of the current quite as much as you lift each foot going forward.

Try to avoid pinch points in a river where the river narrows and water flow is constricted, forcing it to pile up and move faster. Don't even attempt to ford a stream if the current appears too swift or if the depth appears close to being chest deep (the water will always be deeper than you think because of refraction (parallax), a light-bending property). It's not worth the risk. You can toss in a stick to gauge how fast the current is moving where you intend to ford a stream. Pick a spot where the current is relatively slow and does not enter into a funnel before cascading downstream, the depth is less than knee high or waist deep and the substrate is relatively even. You do not want to get your foot jammed amidst large cobble under any circumstances.

Rocks, boulders, fallen trees, etc. all create different levels of friction in a stream. This friction,

Do not be afraid to use a buddy system. If you're small in stature and weight you might want to ask a larger partner to take your hand while fording a stream.

in turn, creates different water surfaces called laminar flows. The basic principle related to laminar flows is that various layers or channels of water move at different speeds. The lower layer of the stream moves more slowly than the top layer, for example. The layers next to the stream bottom and stream banks are the slowest, and each subsequent layer will increase in velocity. The fastest part of the river will be just below the top layer of the river. This means that your feet can have good traction on the stream bottom, but your knees will take the full brunt of the force of the current, which might be so powerful it could knock you over.

Do not be afraid to use a buddy system. If you're small in stature and weight you might want to ask a larger partner to take your hand while fording a stream. As the saying goes, discretion is the better part of valor, and you don't want to go for a swim.

There is also nothing wrong with piggy-backing a person across a stream. I've done this many times with my kids without incident. Don't panic if you fall. While the cold water will be a shock, try to re-gain your footing and head for the nearest shore. It's always a good idea to pack some wind and waterproof matches in the event you need them to dry your clothes or get warm after an accidental bath. Remember to store expensive gear such as cameras in plastic Ziploc bags or other similar waterproof containers in a day pack. Similarly, always keep your pockets zipped shut so object don't fall out should you fall into the water.

Travel on Ice: Lakes, Streams and Rivers

Canadian guidelines regarding travel on ice are similar from one jurisdiction to another. Do not walk on ice that is less than 10 cm (4 inches) thick. Ice thickness should be at least 25 cm (10 inches) for snowmobiles. Don't drive a vehicle on ice that is less than 30 cm (12 inches) thick. Do not travel on ice after dark. Do not take any chances if you are not certain the ice is safe to travel on. Avoid areas where there is visibly open water. However, safety relative to ice thickness is not an exact science, so you should always err on the side of caution when travelling on ice. A number of precautions have already been outlined in a later section, Snowmobile Apparel, Hazards and Travel Guidelines. Personally, when driving in a vehicle on ice, I always travel with the windows rolled at least partially down, and I never lock the doors of a vehicle.

> The Canadian Red Cross recommends the following guidelines respecting danger signals regarding the colour of ice:
>
> 1. The colour of ice may be an indication of its strength.
> 2. Clear blue ice is strongest.
> 3. White opaque or snow ice is half as strong as blue ice. Opaque ice is formed by wet snow freezing on the ice.
> 4. Grey ice is unsafe. The greyness indicates the presence of water.

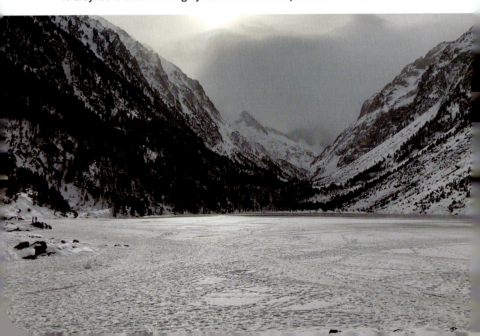

The Canadian Red Cross also recommends the following guidelines (1) when you are alone on ice, and (2) when you are with others on ice.

When You Are Alone on Ice

If you get into trouble on ice and you're by yourself:

- Call for help
- Resist the immediate urge to climb back out where you fell in. The ice is weak in this area
- Try to relax and catch your breath. Turn yourself toward shore so you are looking at where you entered onto the ice. The ice is more stable close to shore
- Reach forward onto the broken ice without pushing down. Kick your legs to try to get your body into a horizonal position
- Continue kicking your legs and crawl onto the ice
- When you are back on the ice, crawl on your stomach or roll away from the open area with your arms and legs spread out as far as possible to evenly distribute your body weight. Do not stand up! Look for shore and make sure you are crawling in the right direction

When You Are with Others on Ice

- Rescuing another person from ice can be dangerous. The safest way to perform a rescue is from shore
- Call for help. Consider whether you can quickly get help from trained professionals (police, fire fighters or ambulance) or bystanders
- Check if you can reach the person using a long pole or branch from shore. If so, lie down and extend the pole to the person
- If you go onto ice, wear a PFD and carry a long pole or branch to test the ice in front of you. Bring something to reach or throw to the person (e.g., pole, weighted rope, line or tree branch)
- When near the break, lie down to distribute your weight and slowly crawl toward the hole
- Remaining low, extend or throw your emergency rescue device (pole, rope, line or branch) to the person
- Have the person kick while you pull them out
- Move the person to a safe position on shore or where you are sure the ice is thick. Signal for help

Caution should always be foremost in the interests of your personal safety. For example, on streams and rivers, the ice thickness often varies depending on the channel and current, with open water sometimes hiding underneath a blanket of snow. Conditions can be especially treacherous below hydropower dams. When travelling on government sanctioned "ice roads," always stay within the bounds, and do not deviate as conditions might be unsafe.

On lakes with heavy snow, overflow can be an issue; it is very easy to get stuck in overflow, which can lead to all sorts of problems, up to and including hypothermia. Areas with overflow are often found near shore and are dangerous as water seeps through cracks to the surface. If you're driving a vehicle

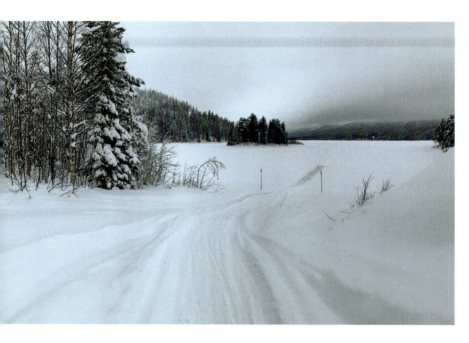

and get stuck, you may have to shovel your way out. Sometimes, by chaining up, you will be able to get free. On rear-wheel drive vehicles, chains should be put on the rear wheels. On 4x4 vehicles, chains should be put on the front tires. It pays to have a buddy system when on the ice so that one vehicle can pull out another if it gets stuck.

Pressure ridges are not uncommon on large lakes and can be an insurmountable obstacle in worst case scenarios. A vehicle causes a shock (pressure) wave to develop in front of it as it travels forward on ice. Consequently, when vehicles are travelling in a convoy, they should stay well apart so as not to intercept a "wave" before it subsides because the ice might be weakened underneath it. This also applies to snowmobiles.

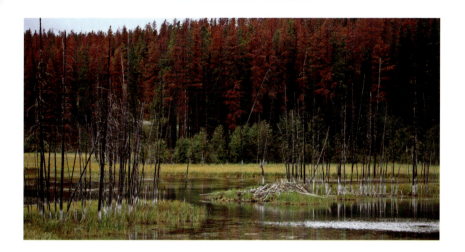

Muskeg

Muskeg (Canadian quicksand): While I've only heard of one example of quicksand in Canada, the Canadian version is more likely in the form of muskeg, which is very common in the boreal forest.

Muskeg (from Cree *maskek* and Ojibwe *mashkiig*, meaning "grassy bog") is a type of northern landscape characterized by a wet environment, vegetation and peat deposits. Muskeg is very common in the boreal forest in western Canada and escapes a precise scientific description. It encompasses various types of wetlands usually associated with a vegetated bog that's made up of moss and other plants, which are saturated with water that can only be safely crossed when frozen. Avoid areas of muskeg as they are very dangerous and can be a death trap. They are plagued with swarms of mosquitoes during the summer.

For a first-hand account of the difficulty of traversing muskeg read R.M. Patterson's The Dangerous River (Chapter 3) for an account between Fort Nelson and Squaw Creek Prairie, British Columbia, on horseback. I had a similar, though relatively minor experience, on a trail ride with my family in the headwaters of the Red Deer River in Alberta, where trails through the muskeg were chest high on our saddle horses. Quite frankly, I thought we were doomed, but the strength and endurance of our horses was incredible as they shouldered their way through the worst patches of muskeg. You did not dare stop or you'd be stuck, so we spurred our mounts until we broke through onto solid ground.

> **Avoid areas of muskeg as they are very dangerous and can be a death trap. They are plagued with swarms of mosquitoes during the summer.**

Preventing Wildlife Encounters

Outdoor travelers should not be afraid to venture into Canada's back country for fear of attacks by wild animals. While bears can be dangerous, it is unlikely they will attack a person if left alone. The same applies to other ungulates and carnivores, but there are always exceptions, so it is best to take a precautionary approach to be on the safe side. If threatened, wild animals will do whatever is necessary to defend themselves or their offspring. Always keep a safe distance from any wild animal as even innocent looking creatures—like a Canadian beaver—will attack a person if they feel threatened.

Do not feed any wild animals. This habituates them to humans and can cause grave problems.

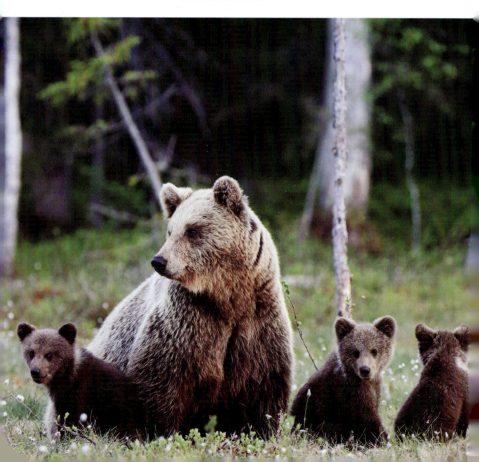

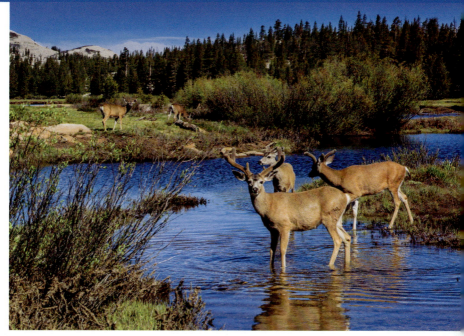
Mule deer

Do not feed any wild animals. This habituates them to humans and can cause grave problems. I once witnessed a woman feeding mule deer in Waterton Lakes National Park in southern Alberta—it is illegal to feed wild animals in Canada's national parks, so she was breaking the law. She had been feeding potato chips to an adult doe and then switched to feed the doe's fawn. The doe reared on its hind legs and raked the woman's face and chest with its front hooves. She suffered serious facial cuts and cuts to her chest and had to be taken to the hospital in Pincher Creek for treatment.

Always keep a clean campsite and store food away from your sleeping area and out of reach of wild animals. Failure to do so might have life-threatening consequences if a bear or wolverine breaks into your food cache and eats everything. Pick up litter that might have been left behind by careless campers and burn table scraps down to ashes so there is no odor to attract bears and other wild creatures.

Always keep a clean campsite and store food away from your sleeping area and out of reach of wild animals.

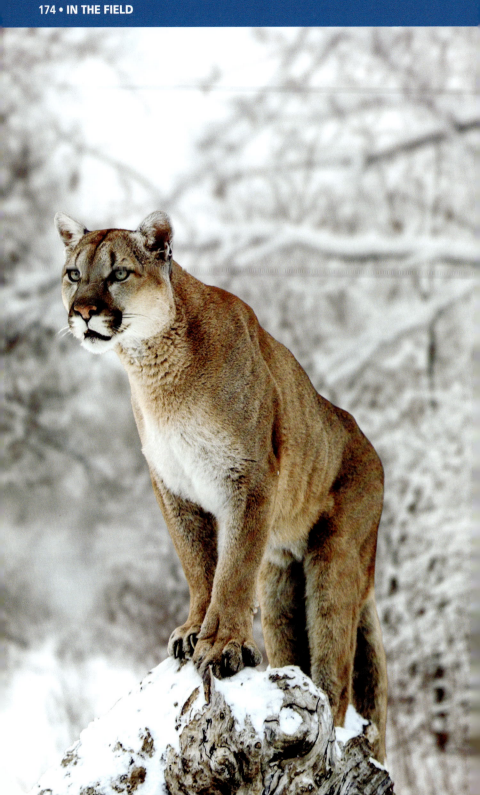

Backcountry Wildlife Safety

My mantra during outdoor excursions is simple: hope for the best and prepare for the worst.

Plan for how you and your party with deal with a crisis. They can, and do, happen to even the most experienced outdoorspeople. Think ahead of time what you will do if you are attacked by a bear or cougar (e.g., what will you do when you realize an attack is imminent?). If you are travelling with other people, make sure you are all on the same page with a contingency plan right down to how to administer first aid if necessary. Every person in your party should have bear spray and bear bangers to try to scare a bear away from camp if needed. In terms of radio communications, my party rented a satellite phone for our Yukon adventure. We knew the phone numbers of the local authorities to call in the case of an emergency. We had a quality first aid kit, and everybody practiced using cans of bear spray and bear bangers. We also had medevac insurance in the event of a worst-case scenario.

Outdoorspeople have good reason to be concerned for their safety in the Canadian outdoors. Hikers, hunters, trappers and prospectors have been mauled and/or killed by black bears, grizzlies and polar bears, cougars, and even coyotes and wolves on rare occasions. For this reason, Inuit hunters are often hired to guard exploration and scientific camps against polar bears.

> If you are travelling with other people, make sure you are all on the same page with a contingency plan right down to how to administer first aid if necessary.

Such attacks often happen without warning or provocation. Sometimes they are predatory in nature (i.e., black bears and cougars), while female grizzlies with cubs may attack people to protect their cubs. Perhaps a person just happens to stumble on a kill site being watched by a nearby grizzly.

The consequences of being attacked by large carnivores in remote areas are particularly problematic—help may be impossible to find, and victims often end up dying from their injuries (in shock) or from hypothermia. While many outdoorspeople carry bear spray and bear bangers, you can't always count on them in an outright attack. When an old friend of mine was attacked by a black bear, he only had time to shoot the bear as it lunged toward him scant yards away. Fortunately for him, he killed it with a single shot.

Bears

The Yukon is Canada's bear capital, so their brochure *How you can stay safe in bear country* is especially instructive: "While there is no guarantee that the advice in this booklet will prevent you from being harmed by a bear, it can help reduce your risks…. If you understand and apply these safety principles, you can make your next trip into bear country safer for both you and the bears." I underscore the same message in this section and provide some tips on how to avoid problem encounters with bears, particularly black bears and grizzlies.

Black bears are present in the forests, foothills and Rocky Mountains in all provinces except Prince Edward Island. Grizzly bears are present in British Columbia and the western boreal forest, foothills and, having recently expanded their range into the short grass prairies, Rocky Mountains in Alberta. Historically, grizzlies were primarily found in the barren grounds of the Northwest Territories and Nunavut but have moved into the Arctic Archipelago over the past decades and are now residents on Victoria Island. Polar

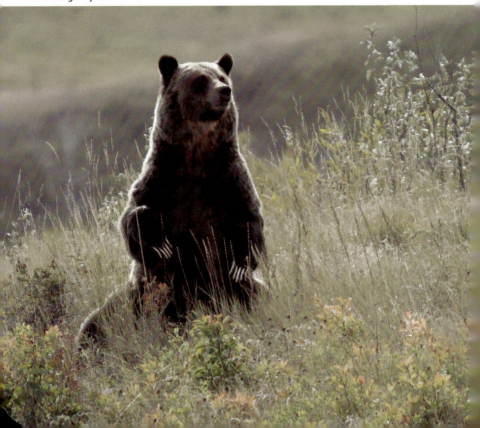

Female grizzly bear

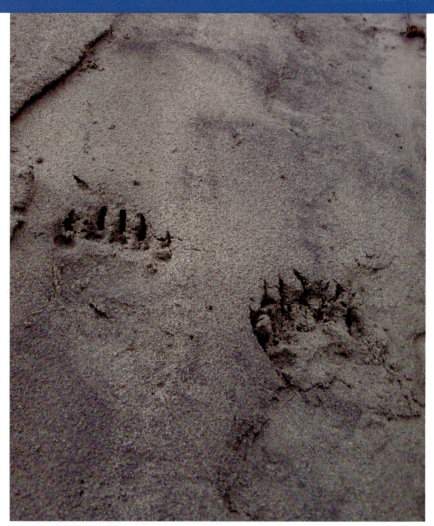
Black bear tracks along the Pitt River, British Columbia.

bears are found throughout the Canadian Arctic (more so in the eastern Arctic), near Churchill in Manitoba, northern Quebec and Labrador.

David O'Farrell of Grizzly Creek Lodge, Yukon says that if a grizzly bear charges within 20 yards, it's best to be prepared for the worst. While most bears will avoid people, there are always exceptions: "A lifetime spent in bear country for many months each year has taught me that the one thing you can count on with bears is that they are incredibly unpredictable," he said in an interview. "You just never know what they will do."

When camping in bear country, the number one safety tip is to keep a clean camp and never eat or store any food in your sleeping tent. This cannot be overstated.

During the late 1960s I worked for the Alberta government doing biological surveys of lakes and streams in the bush in northeastern Alberta. Most of the work required stays at fly-in camps in Canada's remote boreal forest. Black bears were everywhere and were routinely spotted while flying between camps and on lake shores during survey work. One of the first jobs when setting up camp is to dig a pit for garbage, which is burned daily in the evening. In most cases, this was an easy job, except where there was permafrost, such as in the Caribou Mountains, where it could be difficult to find ground that wasn't frozen. But one night, at a camp on Eva Lake, we decided to wait until morning to burn the garbage.

When we awoke around 7:00 AM, I heard the sounds of a bear eating what was left of the garbage in the nearby pit. Normally, the pit would be located some distance from camp, but in this situation, it was hard to find a suitable location because of permafrost. I quietly told my partner, Gordon Bradley, that a bear was near camp. I could see it through a window in the tent, not far away. It was a big, black bear sitting on its haunches and going through the garbage. I dressed quickly and stepped outside with a 12 Gauge shotgun and shouted at the bear, which promptly left. The last thing I wanted to do was shoot the bear, who was just doing what was natural—especially because it was our fault the bear was drawn so close to our camp. After a quick breakfast, we burned all the garbage in the pit and before long a charter float plane arrived to move camp to Pitchimi Lake nearby. I was the crew leader, and it was my job to be the first at a new camp and set up in phases, as it usually took at least a couple of trips to move camp. I left my shotgun with Bradley just in case the black bear showed up again, which it did. Fortunately, it kept its distance, but danced around looking to see what was going on. Gordon held his fire, but was very relieved to get on the float plane and join me at Pitchimi Lake.

We set up an old-fashioned canvas tent for sleeping and a wall tent to store our biological supplies and food, and after dinner we settled into our sleeping bags to the sound of rain on the canvas. Before long, we heard the sound of canvas being torn in the nearby wall tent as a bear tried to get inside. It was pitch dark, raining, with waves lapping on the nearby shore when I stepped out of our tent and yelled at the bear. Thankfully, it took off and didn't return.

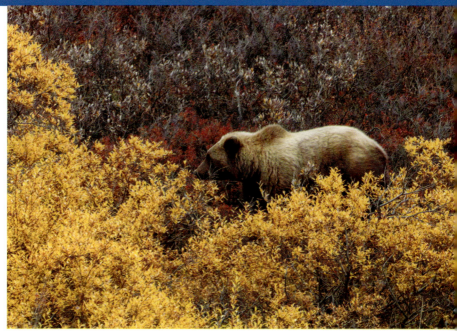

Grizzly bear in fall

Food should be stored in a separate tent or food cache or hung in a tree out of reach of bears—at least 10 feet off the ground.

Arctic authorities recommend solar-powered electric fences and a sentry posted to guard against polar bears. The Trail Riders of the Canadian Rockies have long used electric fences around their teepee camps to keep bears away. I've spent time in their camps in Alberta's Rocky Mountains and never encountered any bears near camp despite bears being in the area.

A person can run into a bear just about any time in the wilderness, except when bears go into a deep sleep during the winter months, known as torpor. However, while bears tend to slow down during the winter, they are not true hibernators, and they have been known to leave their dens during the winter. The autumn is a bit riskier than the other seasons because bears are fattening up, actively feeding in preparation to enter a winter den. They're moving around in search of food, especially ripe berries loaded with sugar such as blueberries,

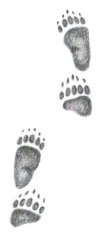

chokecherries, huckleberries and saskatoon berries. These fruit bearing shrubs and bushes are often abundant near creeks and streams where the sound of running water can mask any noises that might alert a bear that humans are nearby—never a good thing.

There is no excuse, however, to let your guard down when you're in the outdoors during other times of the year. One year, while fishing Michel Creek in British Columbia, I rounded a bend in the stream and spotted a dead mule deer doe on an inside bend of the stream that was hung up in a logjam. The doe must have slipped while crossing this notoriously slippery creek, got swept into the log jam and drowned. This situation was hazardous because bears tend to gravitate to valley bottoms in the late summer and would eventually catch wind of the carrion. Grizzlies can smell dead animals from miles away. I made tracks, quick, and got out of the area.

Another danger is inadvertently stumbling across a carcass that a grizzly has found, partially eaten and covered up and is watching from nearby; the bear will probably attack you to protect the carcass. Watch for magpies, crows or ravens that might

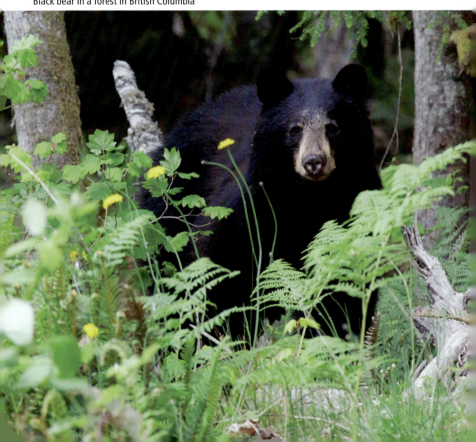

Black bear in a forest in British Columbia

be scavenging a dead carcass. These are all vocal birds, especially in a flock, and you'll often hear them before you see them.

You might find yourself between a sow grizzly and her cubs, in which case the sow will likely attack you to protect her offspring. If you see bear cubs on their own, it is likely the sow is nearby, and you should leave the area immediately.

There are some rare cases when bears will attack unprovoked, such as one involving a hunter who was attacked by a "predatory" grizzly in a remote area near Sundre, Alberta. Black bears have also been known to prey on people; often these animals are emaciated and in poor health. Black bears are notorious for scavenging for food in and around campsites, so it is very important to keep food in a secure location. You should never, under any circumstances, cook any food in your tent when in bear country.

Notwithstanding the foregoing information, I have spent a lifetime in the outdoors, travelling throughout Canada, and I've never had a bad experience with a bear, just some close encounters.

Bears will travel across country over open ground, but where there's

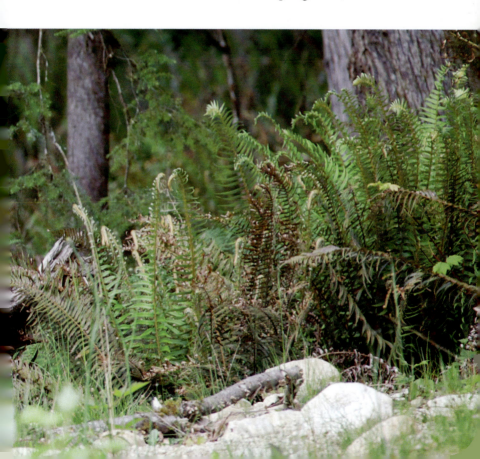

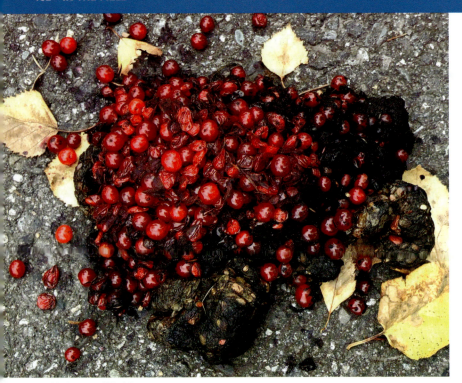

Freshly deposited black bear scat, covered with undigested berries

Always look ahead in your travels; try to spot bears before they spot you, so you don't surprise them. If you do see a bear, do not approach it and give it a wide berth.

bush, they will usually follow game trails. Look for bear scats, which can be distinguished from other carnivore droppings by their sheer size. In the late summer and autumn, bear feces usually have berries in them. If the scats look fresh, be on alert that a bear is nearby.

Black bears will tear up fallen logs and tree stumps in search of insect larva and turn over boulders and rocks for the same purpose. Grizzlies will dig up ground squirrel burrows; these diggings are plainly visible. Grizzlies like to eat the roots of *Hedysarum*, also known as alpine sweet vetch. Watch for bear tracks beside streams and on game trails.

Always look ahead in your travels; try to spot bears before they spot you, so you don't surprise them. If you do see a bear, do not approach it and give it a wide berth.

If you're hiking in bear country, it is a good idea to travel in a group and make some noise to alert bears of your presence. Whenever you are in an area where sight lines are obstructed, repeatedly shout "Yo Bear!" to alert bears that you are nearby so they hopefully move out of the way. The sound of bear bells does not carry far, so they're of little value for making your presence known.

When I'm in bear country, I carry bear bangers as a deterrent that can be launched using a pull-type flare launcher. They make a loud sound when fired and explode at the end of their range. Cracker shells will also work as a deterrent—when fired they make a frightening sound and spiral toward a target, making a screeching noise, before exploding. I've used bear bangers and cracker shells to scare off black bears on coastal streams in British Columbia, and they do work (though I've never tried one on a grizzly). The idea when trying to scare off a bear is to do so while it is still a way off.

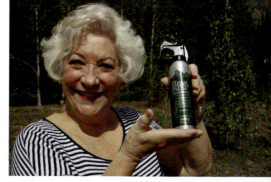

Pack bear spray and practice using it before your trip.

I also carry bear spray, usually two cans if there are grizzlies in the area. There are several types of bear spray on the market. Purchase spray that has a capsaicin concentration of one percent, which is at the upper limit of what is recommended for animals. Capsaicin is a component of chili pepper and is a strong irritant to mammals. Practice using the spray before you venture outdoors, and make sure it has not passed its expiry date. Remember, it won't work in a tent.

Pack bear spray and practice using it before your trip. Also, check the best before date to make sure it has not expired. Purchase spray that has a capsaicin concentration of one percent. You might also want to invest in a holster that can either be worn on your belt or pack strap.

A rule of thumb for bear encounters: If it's black, fight back. If it's brown, lay down. If it's white, say goodnight.

There are no absolute rules regarding what you should do if attacked by a black or grizzly bear. However, consider the following self-defence scenarios that illustrate two fundamental categories of bear attacks.

Provoked Attack

1. You have unintentionally done something that has provoked a bear into showing signs of aggression toward you.

2. It is important that you act passively: de-escalate your posture and do not look directly at the bear. Staring is perceived as aggressive behavior and should be avoided. Always keep the bear in sight so you can flee if necessary. Remember, however, that a human cannot outrun a bear, which can travel at the speed of a racehorse, in short distances (i.e., a grizzly bear can run up to 35 mph in a sprint).

3. If an attack appears imminent, lie down on the ground in the prone position (i.e., play dead) or climb a tree (black bears and some grizzly bears can climb trees, so climbing a tree to try to get out of harm's way is not always an option). These are both signs of submission to the bear and shows the bear that you are no longer a threat to them. Put your hands over your head to protect yourself from the most serious injury.

4. Don't yell at the bear or throw things at them, these are obvious signs of aggression and could further provoke an attack.

Predatory Attack

1. In this case, the bear is obviously hunting or stalking you as potential food. This is a dangerous situation, and you should not "play dead" under these circumstances. Do not try to run away—you will lose the race.

2. You must defend yourself with whatever means are available to save your life. Act aggressively toward the bear: stand up on something high and try to scare it off by making yourself look larger by raising your arms.

3. Try to appear dominant and do whatever you can to try to frighten the bear away. Yell, scream, shout and wave your arms. Jump up and down and fight back. Hold your jacket or backpack over your head to make yourself look bigger.

4. Use your bear defence deterrent to show you mean business; either a bear banger, cracker shell or pepper spray. Bear spray should be used when the bear is within ~3 m or closer to be effective; save it for close quarters.

Polar Bears

If you encounter a polar bear, keep these tips in mind: Try to stay calm and, don't panic; polar bears are fearless and much harder to scare than black bears and grizzlies. Don't act like their prey. Do act like a threat. Use bear spray if threatened. Don't give up if attacked—you'll have to fight for your life. There are no trees to climb on Canada's tundra. Think seriously about being armed with a firearm if travelling in polar bear country or hiring an Inuk guide to act as a guardian. Polar bears are said to be able to run up to 40 mph, so you will never outrun one.

Be proactive and stay safe. Be wary of bears should you recognize signs of their presence nearby and keep your distance should you sight one. Bears are fast, and they can outrun you, so don't take any chances. There are no hard and fast rules when dealing with bear attacks, but prevention is always better than confrontation.

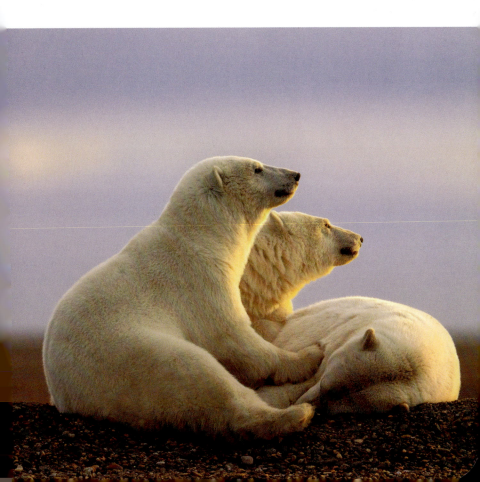

Bison

There are two kinds of bison in Canada: the plains bison and wood bison. The wood bison is much larger than the plains bison, with adult males weighing more than 2,000 pounds. Wood bison are the largest terrestrial animal in North America. Plains bison are a bit smaller, but a big bull could weigh as much as 1900 pounds. Normally, wood bison and plains bison are harmless but cannot always be trusted, especially during the rut in late summer when bulls can be very dangerous.

You should never approach a plains bison or wood bison. Try to give them a wide berth if you see them or encounter them on a forest trail. They are surprising agile on their feet and easy to stampede when alarmed. They are reported to be capable of tops speeds of 65 km/h.

There are an estimated 1,500 to 2,000 plains bison in Canada's national parks, such as Elk Island, Banff, Prince Albert and Waterton Lakes. The bison in Waterton Lakes National Park are in a paddock. Prince Albert National Park in Saskatchewan is home to one of the only free-roaming herds of plains bison on its historic range in Canada, but Parks Canada is in the process of trying to establish a free ranging herd in Banff National Park. Wood Buffalo National Park, which straddles the border between Alberta and the Northwest Territories, is home to Canada's largest herd of wood bison, but it is also common to see them outside of the park, especially in the Northwest Territories. They are also commonly seen along the Alaska Highway in both British Columbia and the Yukon.

If a bison stomps its feet, paws the ground, snorts or starts to hyperventilate, it is likely preparing to charge you, so beware of these warning signs. You will not be able to outrun a bison and may have to climb a tree to avoid being trampled. If you pay attention, however, it is unlikely you will have any misadventures. I've hiked all the trails in Elk Island National Park many times, where both plains and wood bison are numerous, and have never been bothered by them.

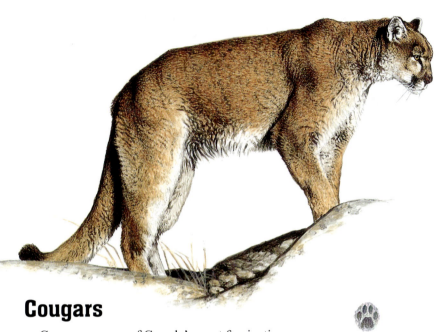

Cougars

Cougars are one of Canada's most fascinating wild creatures. Most of Canada's cougars live in western Canada (primarily in Alberta and British Columbia and are rare in the Yukon) but cougars have also been seen across the prairies, southern Ontario, Québec and New Brunswick. Of the estimated 4000 cougars in Canada, 3500 live in British Columbia. They're majestic predators and powerful enough to bring down large ungulates like bull elk, which can weight over 800 pounds. An adult male cougar can weigh over 220 pounds. They can sprint quickly and outrace their prey but, because they have small lungs, cannot keep up this pace. Cougars can run between 64–80 kms per hour, while a person's top speed is less than 30 kms per hour. It's been said, however, that a person could outrace a cougar in a 100-yard dash. They generally avoid humans and, if threatened, will usually climb a large tree. Normally, they prey on deer and smaller game animals. They are usually found in remote areas and tend to be nocturnal hunters, so they're rarely seen.

If you see a cougar and believe it is acting in a threatening manner, show it that you are not a prey animal and are going to fight back.

In the last 100 years, there have been about 25 fatal cougar attacks in North America, according to the Washington Department of Fish & Wildlife. There has only been one documented death from a cougar attack in Alberta in Banff National Park in 2001. By comparison, five people have been killed by cougar attacks in British Columbia during the past 100 years, all but one of which occurred on Vancouver Island, which has a large population of cougars.

According to Alberta's "Bear Smart" program guidelines, if you see a cougar and believe it is acting in a threatening manner, show it that you are not a prey animal and are going to fight back. Never run. Face the cougar and back away from it, slowly. Shout at the cougar and try to make yourself look bigger than you actually are by waving your arms and opening your jacket to try to intimidate it. Throw rocks or sticks at it. Use a noisemaker or bear spray if it approaches closely. If the cougar attacks, be prepared to use all means at your disposal to fight for your life with a hunting knife, axe, rifle—whatever you have with you, because it probably intends to kill you.

I have been fortunate to have seen three cougars in the wilds of Canada, two of which were stalking mule deer (unsuccessfully) and another wandering in the bush. The largest cougar I've ever seen was taken by hunters in Dutch Creek in southwestern Alberta. It filled the back of a pickup truck—it was that large—and would have weighed more than 200 pounds. There is no way a person could fight off a cougar this large if it decided to attack them, they're simply too big and strong. Fortunately, cougars rarely attack people and usually avoid human contact. However, cougar attacks take place on an irregular basis, often involving children and pets. Often these cougars are young and emaciated, sometimes with a face full of porcupine quills, which would affect their ability to prey on other animals. ❖

Coyotes

There are thousands of coyotes across Canada, almost all of which are completely harmless, but they should always be considered dangerous. For instance, there is a story in the Edmonton Journal (April 24, 2020) about a coyote that attacked a toddler in Coronation Park, at the heart of the city of Edmonton, Alberta—a testament to the need to be careful at all times.

A large, male coyote can weigh up to 45 pounds. They normally feed on rodents, hares, upland game birds, deer, etc. but have been known to attack and kill dogs in and around urban areas. Most coyotes will run away at the first sight of humans, but in recent years, those in and around some Canadian cities are losing their fear of people and coming right into their yards. A couple of years ago, I noticed a coyote eating fallen Hyslop crab-apples in my backyard in Edmonton. I watched it leap on top of my six-foot high fence several times and walk along top of it in search of whatever else might be nearby as a source of food that winter.

There is only been one known human death by coyotes in Canada, which occurred in Nova Scotia's Cape Breton Highlands National Park's Skyline Trail in 2009. At least two coyotes were thought to be involved, although there was a pack of five in the area. It is not unusual for coyotes to gather in a pack in western Canada during the late winter when the snow is deep and prey on large animals like deer.

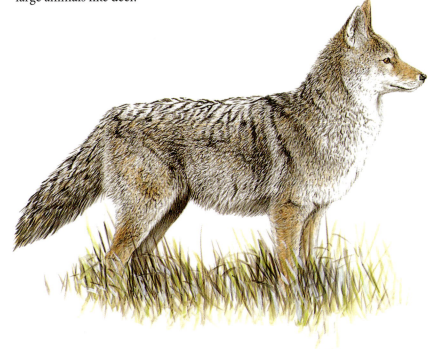

Elk

Elk are large ungulates that are found primarily in British Columbia, Alberta, Saskatchewan and Manitoba, with some also in Ontario. There are more than 72,000 elk in Canada. Those in the wild will almost always flee at the sight of people; however, in Canada's national parks, they have been known to attack people, primarily during the September rutting season. Many wild animals in national parks have lost their fear of people due to habituation and are not to be trusted.

A bull elk will gather in a harem of several—in some cases, up to more than a dozen—cows and defend it against other bulls. The bulls can be very aggressive during the rut and should not be approached under any circumstances at the risk of being gored or trampled. They may attack intruders without warning. A mature bull might weigh anywhere from 700 to 900 pounds and are surprisingly agile and fast on their feet. I am not aware of any human deaths caused by elk in Canada.

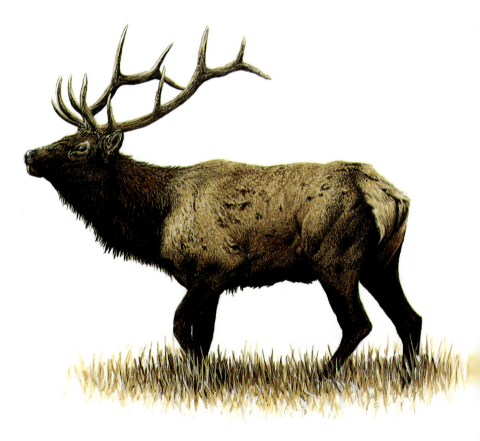

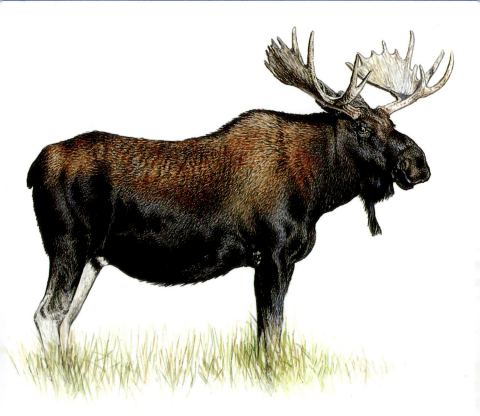

Moose

Moose are present across Canada, except for in the province of Prince Edward Island. There might be up to one million moose in Canada and most are harmless, innocent creatures. They live by their ears and nose but don't see that well, so if you see one and don't want to surprise it, make some noise to get their attention.

There's no such thing as a small moose—cows weigh more than 800 pounds, while males can weigh over 1500 pounds. It is rare for a moose to attack a person unless cornered, but cows with calves should be treated with respect. Never approach a calf moose and never get between a calf moose and its mother. A mother moose will attack a person if it feels the calf is being threatened.

It is not uncommon for cow moose in particular to charge people if they feel threatened, so make sure you do not approach them.

In Canada, hitting a moose or deer with a vehicle is the number one cause of animal deaths. Drive carefully in moose range, and be especially careful during the rut, which occurs in late September–early October, when bulls are most active and on the move.

Wolves

Timber wolves are symbolic of the great outdoors and personify Canada's wilderness. They come in various colours (black, grey and white) and are found across the country, from British Columbia to Labrador, as well as in the Yukon, Northwest Territories and Nunavut, though they aren't found in Prince Edward Island, Newfoundland or Nova Scotia and rarely New Brunswick. They remain one of the most feared and vilified forms of wildlife in Canada. They are often despised by ranchers in western Canada, many of whom would shoot them on sight, because they are known to prey on cattle. Many hunters are upset over wolf predation, especially of elk, bighorn sheep and moose throughout their range. Despite widespread "control" programs in some parts of the country, including bounties and aerial gunning, timber wolf numbers remain high. It is estimated that there are about 60,000 wolves in Canada, and their range is expanding in parts of the country.

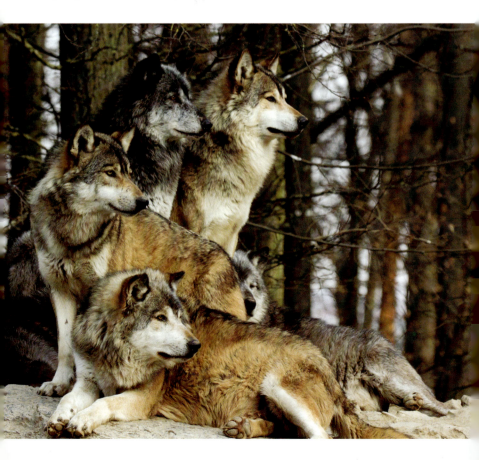

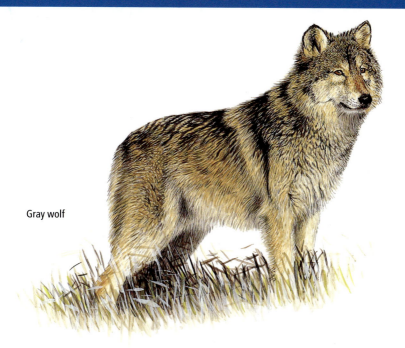

Gray wolf

Most Canadians have never seen a wolf because wolves tend to inhabit remote areas and usually travel in packs; the chances of seeing one are slim when they're bunched together most of the time. The "lone" wolf is rare. My first wolf sighting was that of a huge timber wolf in the Gold Creek Valley, located on Alberta's side of the Crowsnest Pass. It was so big, at first, I thought it was a mule deer. It seemed to vaporize as it quietly slipped away into the forest. Despite having spent a lot of time in Canada's outdoors, I have only seen about a dozen gray wolves in my lifetime in the Elk Valley in British Columbia, along the continental divide between Alberta and British Columbia near Phillip's Pass, in Jasper National Park and throughout the boreal forest and Canadian Shield in northern Alberta. Even though I have made about 20 backcountry trips in remote areas of the Yukon, Northwest Territories and Nunavut, I've yet to see any wolves there.

There is a lot of unsubstantiated, sensational online information about timber wolves in Canada regarding their status and behavior, so take it with a grain of salt. Ted Lyon and Will Graves, the authors of *The Real Wolf, The Science, Politics, and Economics of Co-Existing with Wolves in Modern Times* debunked the popular public misconception that wolves are relatively benign, shy creatures that do not harm people, when in fact they have killed many people (especially in Europe), as well as pets and livestock. Regardless, there have been only two verified fatal healthy (wild) wolf attacks on humans in North America, one of which was at Points North Landing in northern Saskatchewan in 2005.

Outdoorspeople usually have little to fear from wolves in Canada. Most wolves would flee at the sight of a person. However, there are always exceptions, so you can never be too careful. For instance, in Banff National Park in 2019, a family of four was attacked by a wolf while they slept. While Parks Canada officials said that incidents such as this one are extremely rare in Banff National Park, there have been other wolf attacks in provincial parks in British Columbia and Ontario. Take whatever measures you can to ward of an attack by a wolf, which are very strong and fully capable of killing a person. The best advice I can give if you are attacked by a wolf is to fight for your life.

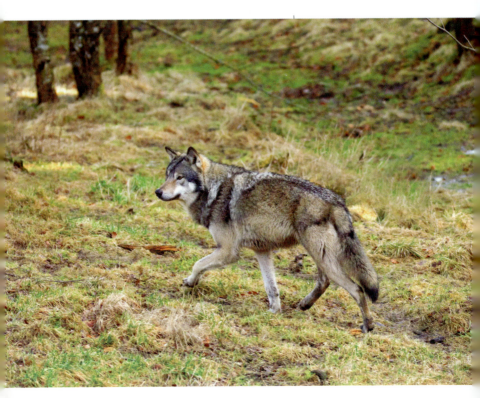

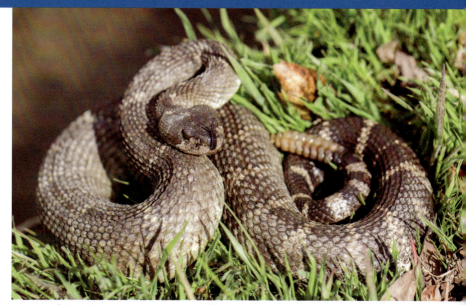
Northern pacific rattlesnake

Snakes

There have only been a few recorded deaths from snakes in all of Canada because most species of snakes in Canada are non-venomous, non-aggressive and harmless if left alone. They are generally quite shy. As reptiles, they are cold blooded animals and are inactive when temperatures are cold. In the autumn, they move into a hibernaculum where they overwinter. I've only stumbled across one hibernaculum of garter snakes beside the Crowsnest River in southern Alberta, which was quite an education. Dozens of garter snakes were denned up underneath a sandstone ledge amongst a boulder pile and curled up in tight ball. Snakes will normally flee from a person, with the possible exception of bull snakes. Bull snakes are large reptiles found in western Canada that may act aggressively if threatened. They will hiss and may even strike out at a person if disturbed, so they should be left alone. Snakes are found in all Canadian provinces, except Newfoundland, as far north as Wood Buffalo National Park in the Northwest Territories.

Snakes are found in all Canadian provinces, except Newfoundland, as far north as Wood Buffalo National Park in the Northwest Territories.

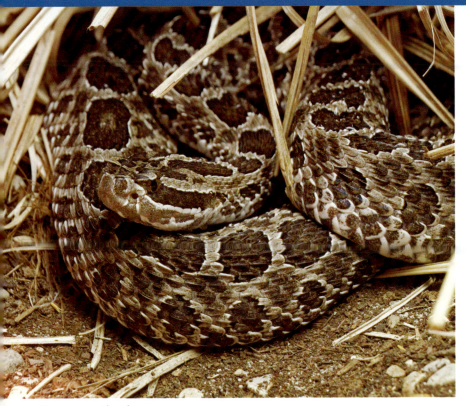

Massasauga rattlesnake

According to the Canadian Wildlife Federation, the following dangerous, venomous snakes can be found in Canada:

1. **Northern Pacific Rattlesnake** (*Crotalus oreganus oreganus*), a subspecies of the Western Rattlesnake: This snake is found in the interior of British Columbia and can measure more than 1.5 m in length. The British Columbia population is small and confined to dry grasslands in bunchgrass and ponderosa pine zones of Okanagan-Similkameen, Thompson, Nicola and Kettle valleys, as well as the Lytton-Lillooet portion of the Fraser Canyon. They prefer short-grass prairie and dry, open scrubland. When disturbed, like other rattlesnakes, they defend themselves by coiling, vibrating their rattle and striking. While their bites are seldom fatal, you should always be cautious when around these snakes.

2. **Massasauga Rattlesnake** *(Sistrurus catenatus):* These snakes are found primarily around the Georgian Bay area on Lake Huron in Ontario. They seldom grow longer than 75 cm and are commonly found near water. They are not an aggressive creature by nature and will often remain motionless unless disturbed. However, they will coil and can strike if they feel threatened. They can deliver a fatal bite.

3. **Desert Nightsnake** *(Hypsiglena torquata):* The range of this species is confined to a small portion of southern British Columbia in the southern Okanagan and the Lower Similkameen Valley. It measures between about 25–50 cm in length. They like hot, dry areas and are active mainly at night and, consequently, seldom seen. Their saliva is slightly toxic, so take precautions if you happen upon one.

4. **Prairie (western) rattlesnake** *(Crotalus oreganus):* These snakes are found in southern Saskatchewan and Alberta usually in native grasslands in and around major rivers such as the Milk, Oldman, Red Deer and South Saskatchewan. Prairie rattlesnakes can reach a maximum length of 1.5 m. They prefer short-grass prairie and dry, open scrubland. If disturbed, they will defend themselves by coiling, vibrating their rattle and striking. While their strikes are seldom fatal, they are venomous, and you should be careful when you are around them. In my experience, the sound of their rattle is soft and difficult to pick up if there is any amount of wind, which is almost a constant in southern Alberta and Saskatchewan. If you see a rattlesnake or hear a rattle, you should stop and slowly back away out of the danger zone and give the snake a wide berth.

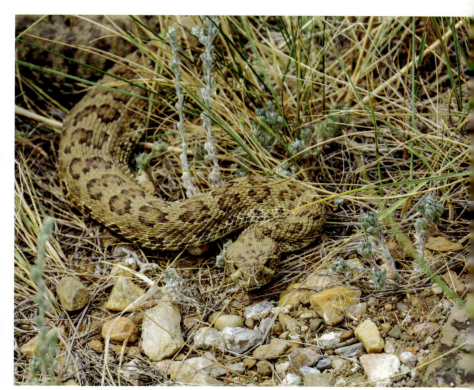

Prairie (western) rattlesnake

Especially hazardous areas are located around abandoned farm buildings, field stone piled around fence posts, at gates, on barb wire fences and elsewhere in pastures, plus rocky outcrops in river valleys where they like to sun themselves. They have been known to enter tents along the Milk River, so make sure the entrances are closed at all times. A person would usually have to search out a prairie rattlesnake to find one because they are rare and live a reclusive life in rugged, uninhabited areas. That being said, they have also been known to come into major urban centres in southern Alberta, such as Lethbridge and Medicine Hat, in search of prey and shelter. One of the most interesting experiences I've ever had was when I chanced upon a female prairie rattlesnake with her offspring not far from the banks of the Milk River in southern Alberta. Rattlesnakes are viviparous and this female had over a dozen pencil sized offspring lying beside her when I walked by her den.

All rattlesnakes and the Desert Nightsnake are protected in Canada and it is illegal to harm, kill, or capture them.

Tips to Avoid Snake Bites

The Ontario Poison Centre offers practical guidelines regarding (1) tips to avoid snake bites, (2) first aid for snake bites if bitten by an unknown or non-venomous snake and (3) what you should not do. I have adapted these guidelines, as well as guidelines from Alberta and British Columbia, as follows:

> **Especially hazardous areas are located around abandoned farm buildings, field stone piled around fence posts, at gates, on barb wire fences and elsewhere in pastures, plus rocky outcrops in river valleys where snakes like to sun themselves**

1. Wear hiking boots and long pants when walking in long grass or rocky areas, especially in places where rattlesnakes are known to live.
2. Watch where you are walking. Do not reach into areas that you cannot see.
3. Be very careful when hiking at night, and use a flashlight to spot any snakes on a trail or at a campsite.
4. If you hear a rattle, stop and listen. Slowly move away from the sound of the snake. Do not try to touch it. The snake will try to move away from you or remain in the same place.
5. Remember it is against the law to kill or harm rattlesnakes in Canada.

Insects

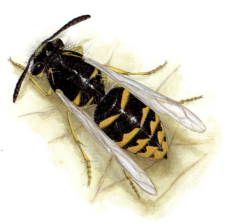

There are no scorpions or tarantulas in Canada, but there are lots of bad insects and bugs. The worst species of insects in Canada's outdoors are mosquitos, black flies, horseflies, deer flies, no-se-ums, hornets and yellow-jacket wasps (sometimes bees if their nests are disturbed), in no particular order. Most insect repellents contain diethyltoluamide (DEET). DEET is a colorless liquid that has a faint odor and does not dissolve easily in water that was developed by the U.S. Army in 1946 for protecting soldiers in insect-infested areas. Most sources indicate that products with concentrations around 10 percent DEET are effective for periods of approximately two hours. As the concentration of DEET increases, the duration of protection increases. For example, a DEET concentration of about 24 percent has been shown to provide an average of five hours of protection. Cigar, cigarette and pipe smoke will repel mosquitoes as well as campfire smudges. If you are ever stranded in the wild, a campfire smudge will provide much needed protection as well as a signal for search and rescue officials.

Insects can be a plague particularly in northern Canada, especially in the boreal forest and barren lands, but not necessarily in Yukon because most of this territory is actually quite dry. I've travelled from coast to coast to coast, and the worst places I have seen for mosquitos were in the Northern Peninsula of Newfoundland and the shortgrass prairies near Brooks, Alberta, of all places. The abundance of mosquitos is closely related to local precipitation as they lay their eggs in ponds and stagnant water. Mosquitos are often at their worst just before a storm.

I have seen insects drive some people practically nuts—especially blackflies as it appears that there is no repellant that works effectively against these biting insects (repellents that are formulated with a 25 percent DEET are of some help though). I've seen men who worked in the boreal forest near Fort Smith, Northwest Territories, bleeding profusely from hundreds of blackfly bites, especially around the wrists, waist, ankles, face and neck. Getting an infection is a serious issue in such cases.

Some people have allergic reactions to the sting of bees and wasps, which can be deadly. If a person is susceptible to an allergic reaction to insect bites, they should carry an epinephrine autoinjector (EpiPen, Auvi-Q, others) to treat an allergic attack.

Contrary to some research findings, I have always found that citronella candles effectively repel mosquitos, reducing the number of mosquitos around them. In fact, I have watched them fly away from the citronella smoke many times. Apparently, citronella also works by masking scents that are attractive to insects, namely carbon dioxide and lactic acid in humans. Mosquitos can follow a trail of carbon dioxide from a person's breath, which seems to be masked by the smoke.

Experienced outdoorspeople will also search out campsites on high, dry ground in the open where there is a breeze to lessen chances of biting insects being a nuisance. Mosquitos are also attracted to people who wear dark clothing, so it is best to wear light-coloured long pants and shirts as well as a hat at all times. If a person is really bothered by biting insects, they should use a mosquito bar when sleeping and wear a mosquito head net hat. Spray the area inside the mosquito bar with an insect pesticide before retiring. I purchased a head net many years ago during a trip to Awesome Lake, Labrador but never used it. Though as a precaution, I have always taken the head net with me across Canada just in case I encounter conditions that are not bearable.

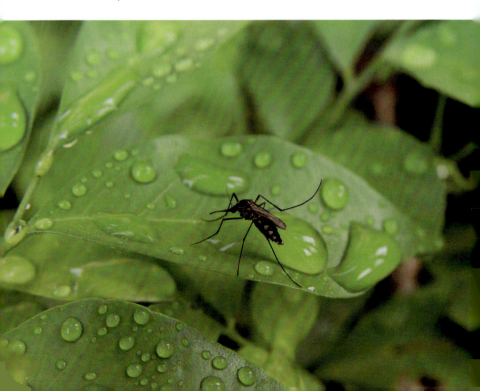

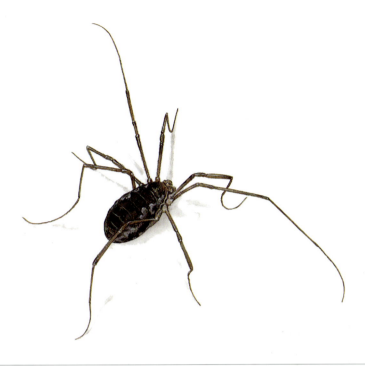

Spiders

There are a few poisonous spiders that are native to Canada, but of greater concern are spider bites that can cause life-threatening blood infections, so any spider bite should be treated with extreme caution. There is the black widow spider, of which there are two species: the western black widow, found in parts of British Columbia through to Manitoba (mostly restricted to areas close to the southern Canada–U.S. border), and the northern black widow in southern and eastern Ontario. In my experience in southern Alberta, I have found black widow spiders are rare; they're shy and will not bother you if you don't bother them. The brown recluse spider, also known as the Fiddleback spider, are not as aggressive as the black widow spiders and will only bite if they are aggravated. They are mostly found in British Columbia, though there have been reports of brown recluse spiders in southern Ontario.

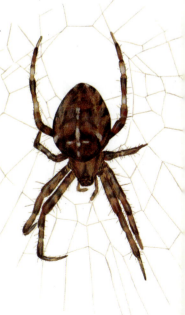

Wood Ticks and Related Diseases

Wood ticks are common throughout Canada and are of particular concern because they can spread diseases that can be fatal. Most people pick up ticks when walking through grass and shrubs. The ticks become dislodged and find a purchase on people. It is a good idea to check your clothing (frequently) when walking outdoors. Denim and cotton garments are probably the worst types of fabric that you can wear as ticks can easily adhere to them. In my experience, and according to outdoor lore, ticks usually travel to a person's armpit, head or groin where it's warm. So, if you feel something crawling on your arm, leg or neck stop and look for a tick. They will eventually try to insert their mouth into your skin and gorge themselves with blood.

Do not try to remove ticks by hand or with forceps if they've inserted their mouth into your skin. Use a heated needle to get them to back out on their own to prevent infections. I've found dozens of ticks on my pant legs after hiking in Alberta's Crowsnest Pass area, as well as on my neck and in my hair. Also, be sure to always check your pets for ticks after taking them on walks in the outdoors.

Medical authorities agree that Lyme disease, caused by *Borrelia burgdorferi* bacteria harbored and spread through the bite of infected ticks, is becoming more common in Canada. In 2015, there were more than 700 cases of Lyme disease reported to the Public Health Agency of Canada, up from roughly 130 in 2009. The Canadian range of Lyme disease is expanding, and it is currently endemic in areas of six provinces: British Columbia, Manitoba, Ontario, Quebec, New Brunswick and Nova Scotia.

Rocky Mountain spotted fever (RMSF) is a bacterial infection spread by a bite from an infected tick, *Dermacentor variabilis*. It is also called tick fever, spotted fever or tick typhus. It causes vomiting, a sudden high fever around 38°C or 39°C (102°F or 103°F), headache, nausea, chills, abdominal pain, a body rash and a severe headache and muscle aches. According to the Mayo Clinic, "Without prompt treatment, Rocky Mountain spotted fever can cause serious damage to internal organs, such as your kidneys and heart." Although many people become ill within the first week after infection, signs and symptoms may not appear for up to 14 days. Fortunately, RMSF has a low incidence in Canada.

Other Diseases

Canada does not have endemic world health diseases like *Dengue fever*, Ebola, HIV/AIDS OR malaria. Fortunately, other outdoor related diseases in Canada are relatively rare, but they can occur, such as Giardiasis (beaver fever), rabies and Trichinosis (caused by a parasite) and West Nile Virus, some of which are deadly.

Giardiasis (an infection of the small intestine), commonly known as beaver fever, is actually a parasitic disease caused by *Giardia duodenalis*, a microscopic parasite (a protozoan flagellate) found in water and most likely infected by rodent feces. Sources indicate that about 10% of those infected have no symptoms. When symptoms do occur, they may include diarrhea, abdominal pain and weight loss. A friend of mine developed beaver fever after drinking water from a mountain stream that I would have considered a pure source of water. He was very sick for several days, with an upset stomach, diarrhea and a lack of an appetite. This illustrates the need to purify drinking water, even if you think it is from a pure source.

Rabies is a fatal viral infection which spreads when a dog is bitten by an infected animal. If your dog gnaws or fixates on the bite mark, or shows signs of irritability or restlessness, these could be symptoms. Fortunately, human rabies is rare in Canada, although it has been detected in several provinces and more commonly found in Ontario and Quebec. Nowadays, it is most commonly spread by rabid bats, but it has also been found in racoons, skunks and red and Arctic foxes.

Trichinosis is a parasitic disease caused by roundworms of the *Trichinella* genus. During the initial infection, invasion of the intestines can result in diarrhea, abdominal pain and vomiting. In Canada, the *Trichinella* roundworm is commonly found in wild bears and foxes. It is transmitted to humans who eat raw or undercooked meat from an animal infected with *Trichinella*. Do not eat raw or undercooked meat to prevent infections.

Sources indicate that in 2002, Canada had its first confirmed human cases of West Nile virus in parts of Quebec and Ontario. That year, 426 Canadians became ill after being infected with the virus. Most people infected with West Nile virus show mild flu-like symptoms or no symptoms at all. Mild signs and symptoms of a West Nile virus infection generally go away on their own. But severe signs and symptoms, such as a severe headache, fever, disorientation or sudden weakness, require immediate attention. Exposure to mosquitoes where West Nile virus exists increases your risk of getting infected.

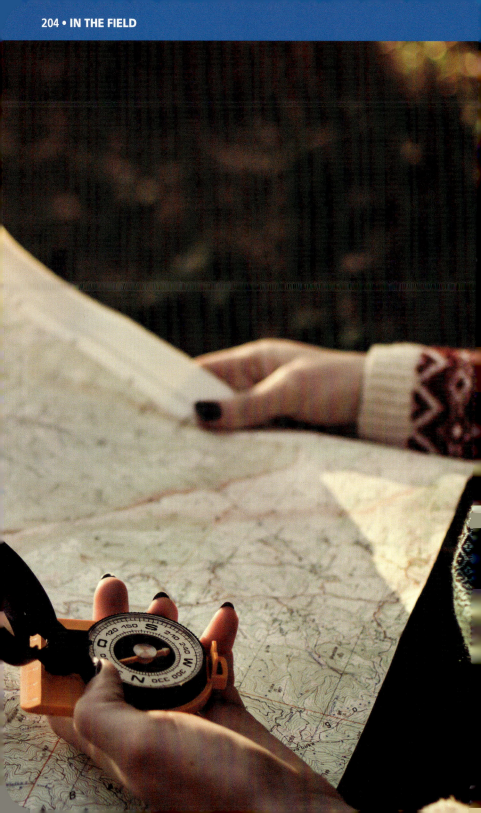

Navigation

Getting lost in the wild is always an issue of concern and rightly so. Anybody can get disoriented and lose their bearings, even experienced outdoorspeople, particularly when skies are overcast, it is snowing, the land is unbroken—land that appears featureless—and where landmarks aren't obvious.

With a Compass

When out on outdoor trips, I make it a point to carry a compass to check my bearings so I can find my way back to camp should I become disoriented. In all cases, a compass works best to orient yourself relative to a topographic map. You will know where you are at the start of the day (your starting point is called a "trailhead"). You can then plot the direction you intend to take based on the topographic map. The "needle" of the compass will point to the magnetic north. You can take a bearing to your destination by aligning the "direction of travel arrow" on the map with the "orienting arrow" on your compass and stay on this bearing until you reach your destination. This is where a compass comes in handy—by making walking in a straight line possible.

A compass works best to orient yourself relative to a topographic map.

Without a Compass

Sun

You can also use the position of the sun to guide you. In the northern hemisphere, if you're travelling north, your shadow will be on your left side; if you're travelling south, your shadow will be on your right side. Let's say you're travelling west in the morning—the sun will be at your back and your shadow in front of you. Remember, however, that in northern latitudes in the autumn and winter, the sun will be lower on the horizon than it will be in the spring and the summer.

In the northern hemisphere, if you're travelling north, your shadow will be on your left; if you're travelling south, your shadow will be on your right.

Celestial Navigation

To find your direction at night without a compass or GPS, you can check out the location of "Venus." Venus, known as the "morning star" and the "evening star," shines brightly in the southwestern skies in Canada. The North Star, also known as Polaris, stays fixed in sky in the northern hemisphere, and it marks the location of the (sky's) north pole. Use the Big Dipper to find Polaris: a line from the two outermost *stars* in the bowl of the Big Dipper points to Polaris; Polaris marks the tip of the handle of the Little Dipper.

Other Methods

It is important to mentally mark key landmarks when travelling in the outdoors so you don't get mixed up. I always make a point of stopping from time to time to check my backtrack so that the landscape doesn't look strange if I have to turn around and head back to the trailhead.

Daytime Navigation: The "Shadow" Method

If you don't have a compass or GPS unit and need to find true north during the day, you can use the "shadow" method. This method is best done on level ground when skies are clear.

1. Stand a straight stick up in the ground and mark where the stick's shadow lands (e.g. with a rock); this mark represents west.

2. Repeat this measurement again after 15–30 minutes. Then, mark the shadow's new location; this mark represents east.

3. Draw a line between the two marks, and stand in front of the line (the first mark, west, should be on your left, and the second mark, east, should be on your right).

4. When you stand in front of the line running from east to west, north will be in front of you and south behind you.

Knots

While there are dozens of different knots used for various purposes only a few key knots are important for survival purposes. There are online diagrams and videos that illustrate how these key knots are tied which can be difficult to describe in words.

Bow Knot

The bow knot has been called the most useful knot in the world. It is also called a bowline knot and is used to make a fixed loop at the end of a rope.

(1) Lay the rope across your left hand with the free end hanging down. Make a small loop in the line in your hand. (2) Bring the free end up and pass it through the eye from the under side of the rope. (3) Wrap the line around the standing line and back down through the loop. (4) Tighten the knot by pulling on the free end while holding the standing rope.

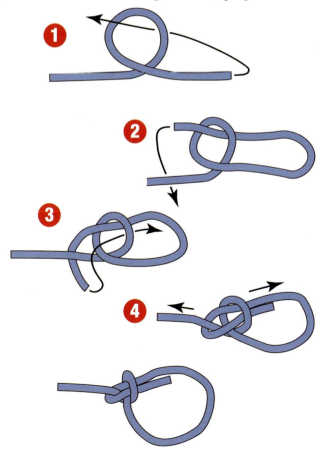

Half Hitch

The half hitch is used to tie rope around an object and back to itself.

(1) Form a loop around the object. (2) Pass the end around the standing end and through the loop. (3) Tighten into a "half hitch" which is designed to secure a load on the standing end. The first half hitch knot is usually followed by a second—or more—half hitch to make certain the knot won't slip.

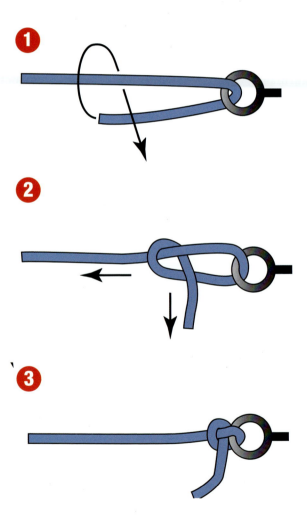

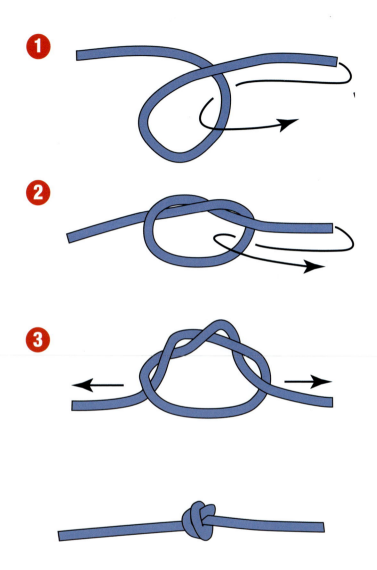

Overhand Knot

A simple "stopper knot" that will prevent the end of a rope from unravelling.

(1) Form a loop and pass the end of the rope through it. (2) Tighten the loop to form the "overhand" knot. (3) Pull the knot tight so it functions as a simple stopper knot.

Slip Knot

A *slip knot* forms an adjustable loop or noose at the end or middle of a rope. (1) Make a loop in the end of a rope by doubling line back onto itself. (2) Run the tag end back towards the loop and lay it over the doubled lines. (3) Make one (or two) turns with the tag end around the doubled lines and through the new loop. (4) Tighten the knot to make it secure.

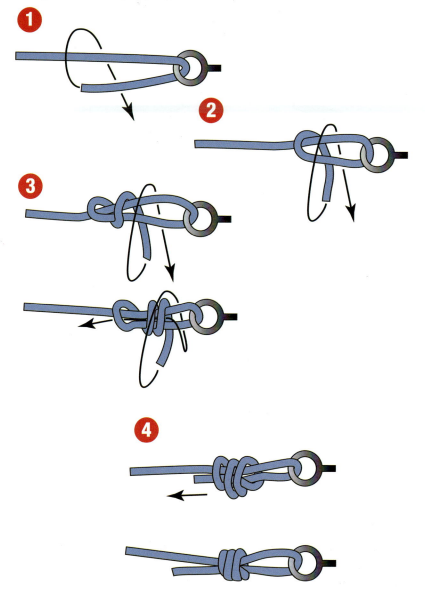

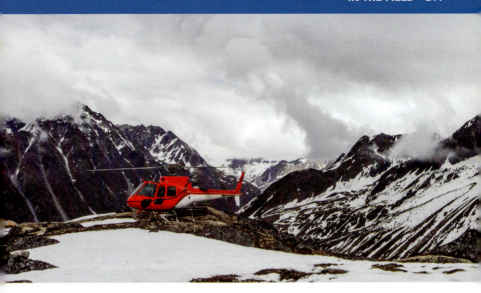

How to Be Found

Canada's Search and Rescue Operations: In Canada, search and rescue (SAR) is a shared responsibility under a National Search and Rescue Program. Many partners are involved because of Canada's immense size, range of terrain and weather. Partners consist of government, military, volunteer and industry groups. They all work together to provide SAR services across the nation. Canadian Armed Forces SAR crews are on standby 24 hours a day, 7 days a week and headquartered in Western, Central, Eastern and Northern Canada.

It's important for people to act responsibly and take safety precautions when in the outdoors, because if they don't follow due diligence, they may have to bear the rescue costs.

For example, when a group of four young men, who knowingly went into an out of bounds area at British Columbia's Grouse Mountain Resort, "freely admitted what they did was wrong," there were financial consequences. They were also "stripped of their passes, banned for life from the resort, and told they would be responsible for the cost of the helicopter flight as well as the resources diverted from the rest of the mountain during their rescue."

In most cases, people who have been rescued from outdoor misadventures will be admitted to a hospital for observation. If medical attention is necessary, the normal treatment procedures will be followed for such things as burns, concussions, fractures, heat stroke, hypothermia, sprains, and so on. Generally, these costs are covered by universal Medicare for Canadians. Healthcare in Canada is delivered through the provincial and territorial systems of publicly funded health care, informally called Medicare. Non-Canadians travelling in Canada should have medical and travel insurance.

Signalling

Best Places to Be Seen

The best places to be spotted by a search party are in open areas, such as forest clearings, ridge tops and beaches on lakes or spits on streams where you'll be visible.

Smoke Signalling

Fires have long been used to signal for assistance or help in Canada's bush country.

Once a fire is started, add some evergreen branches to create smoke to attract attention of passerby or aircraft. If you are stranded, have all the materials necessary for a signal fire on the ready.

Many years ago, while taking biological surveys of lakes and streams in northern Alberta, my crew was camped at an unnamed fly-in lake in the boreal forest and were expecting a charter flight to arrive in the morning to move camp to another lake. The pilot, however, was acting in relief of the pilot who usually flew the charter flight. The pilot didn't know where our camp was located on this large, unnamed lake and perhaps had second thoughts whether this was even the lake we were camped on. We had all of our gear packed and ready to move,

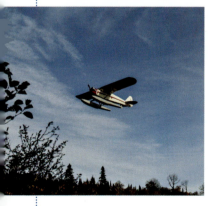

but we left our tent standing, as is the normal practice when flying charter flights, just in case they don't show. We saw the plane on the horizon, and it circled the lake looking for our camp, twice. It was obvious the pilot couldn't locate our camp. I was convinced that he would head back to his base after a third fly over if he didn't spot us. We were low on grub and needed a re-supply, and there was no telling when he'd return. Because our usual pilot would be out of the country, there was an outside chance that we'd be left stranded.

As a last resort, I opened an outboard motor fuel tank and doused a small spruce tree on the shore of the lake with fuel and torched it. The tree burst into flame with lots of smoke. The pilot spotted the smoke, rocked (waggled) the plane's wings to signal that he had seen us and banked the float plane in our direction. After he landed, he told us that if we hadn't signaled him, he would have went back to Fort Chipewyan, Alberta. We put the fire out with some lake water and thanked our lucky stars.

Whistles

It is a good idea to carry a whistle with you in case you need to signal for help. There are many whistles on the market. Pick one that you feel comfortable using.

Forget about Morse code as a basic signal; I find it too complicated. Rather, I suggest that outdoorspeople adopt the "International Whistle Codes" for survival purposes.

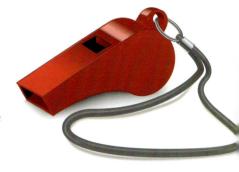

Three blasts of the whistle are an international distress call, which is loosely translated to "Help me!" or "SOS." Two blasts of the whistle are a call-back signal which means "Come here." One blast can mean "Where are you?" or it can be a call-back signal if you hear anything that sounds like a code. Ideally, each whistle blast should last three seconds.

One Blast =	Where are you? OR Call-back signal
Two Blasts =	Come here.
Three Blasts =	Help me! OR SO

Note: The international distress call (three blasts of the whistle) can be made by any noise in groups of three, such as three consecutive bangs of a stick against a tree or other object.

Car Survival

If you get stranded in a vehicle, it's usually best to stay in the vehicle until help arrives, so it's key to be prepared for such emergencies. You will have to try to stay warm so you don't freeze to death under such conditions. Make sure you have adequate clothing for the weather conditions before you leave home. Leave a window slightly open if you are worried about air supply.

Canadian motorists realize that winter is a fact of life, lasting upwards of 6+ months with temperatures reaching extreme conditions in many parts of the country. The temperatures are usually lowest in the months of January and February. It's not just the northern parts of the country that see extremely low temperatures. In Edmonton, Alberta, February, 2019 was one of the coldest months in its history. The mean temperature for this month was −19.4°C, and extreme cold warnings were in place in Edmonton for 14 of 28 days. The following year, on January 15, 2020, the temperature plunged to −37.8°C, the *coldest temperature* in *Edmonton* since it hit −37.8°C on January 19, 1996. The *record* low for January 15 in Edmonton is −43.9°C, set in 1896.

Because of cold temperatures, travel in vehicles can be dangerous, especially in remote areas of northern Canada, northern Ontario, Quebec and Labrador, where hundreds of miles of unpaved roads are still common in the mountains, boreal forest and Pre-Cambrian Shield and throughout the prairie provinces. Winter tires are necessary, which have better traction on snow and ice than summer tires. Often, travel in 4x4 vehicles is recommended. Block heaters should be plugged in overnight when the temperature falls below −15°C. Tire pressure should be increased to compensate for cold temperatures. The Canadian Motor Association recommends motorists have emergency kits in the event of vehicle breakdowns. When temperatures drop below 0°C, parts tend to seize or break, and older vehicles are particularly susceptible to mechanical breakdowns.

It is not unusual for the thermostat to fail during cold weather. Some signs of a faulty thermostat are coolant leaks under the vehicle, engine overheating and high engine temperature readings if the thermostat is stuck or the vehicle will not warm up and the heater will blow cold air. Old batteries can fail, and,

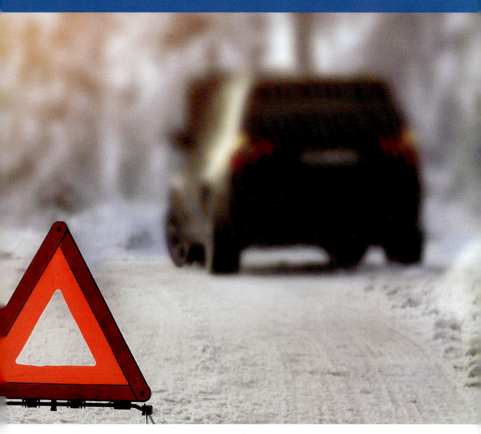

when this happens, the battery must be heated inside a building as a last resort to try to start motors. Your battery should be tested before departing on road trips to ensure it's up to strength.

In case of a breakdown, it is a good idea to have an emergency kit in your vehicle (see Survival Kits on page 38).

Here are some additional winter driving tips based on my personal experience:

- Check your brakes before heading out.
- Knock off any snow and ice from the inside of your wheels to maintain their balance.
- Drive with enough speed to break through hard, crusted drifts on backcountry trails.

Bring a portable battery booster in case your battery fails and a portable compressor in case you need some added tire pressure. Be sure to top off your gas tank when travelling in rural Canada. If there are power outages, you won't be able to gas up. Keep at least half a tank of gas, and try to keep the tank full to minimize condensation.

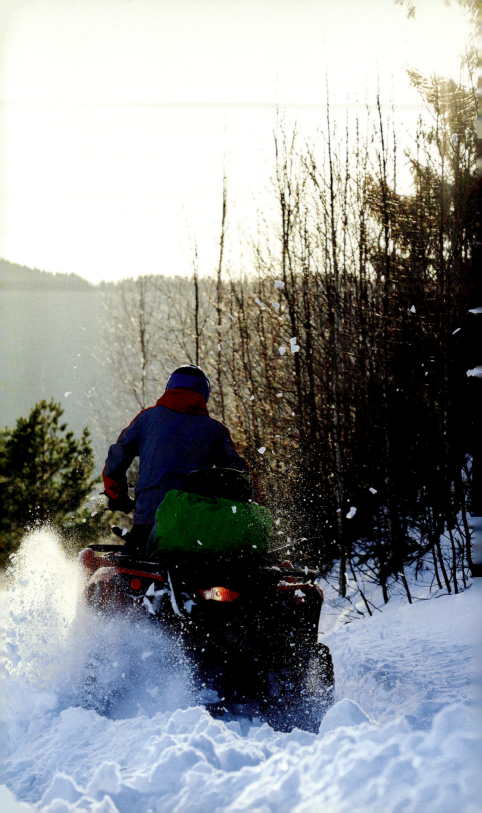

SECTION 3
Specialized Outdoor Activities

⋊•◦●◦•⋉

Boat Safety and Troubleshooting

The D.R. (The Dangerous River) tells of trips made in the North just before the aeroplane made all places accessible to any kind of man, however soft he might be and however useless in the bush. Those of us who had the good fortune to be on the South Nahanni [Northwest Territories] in those last days of the old North may, in times of hunger and hardship, have cursed the day we ever heart the name of that fabled river.

by R. M. Patterson, author, 1966

The Dangerous River is an entertaining novel primarily about the author, R. M. Patterson, and a friend of his named Gordon Matthews, who ventured into the Nahanni River, before this storied area was accessible, to prospect (for gold) and trap furs in the late 1920s. The book stands testament to survival skills associated with treacherous northern rivers, dated though they might be, because they're just as relevant nowadays as ever. *The Dangerous River* remains a classic novel in the genre of Canadian outdoor survival challenges. The author, of British origin, was not an experienced outdoorsman, but he was a very capable person with a lot of imagination and life skills. I'd put him in the category of an "adventurer," who was a greenhorn in many ways. It is amazing he wasn't killed as a result of a misadventure.

In the book's Epilogue by Janet (Patterson) Blanchet (the author's daughter) she says, "To see the canyons of the Nahanni is to marvel at R.M.P.'s journey upstream, alone, inexperienced, paddling or tracking a loaded, sixteen-foot canoe. Given the vertical walls of those canyons, such a venture appears absolutely impossible. Fortunately, R.M.P. was a very lucky man."

Legal Requirements and Life-Saving Appliances

The single most important thing that one can do to prevent drowning is to always wear a properly adjusted PFD or lifejacket of appropriate type, size and fit when on the water.

Transport Canada requires that all operators of motorboats and other powered watercraft take an approved "Boating Safety Course" and obtain a "Pleasure Craft Operator Card." The course material can be studied online before taking a test. By law, effective April 15, 2011, boaters of all ages (there are no age exemptions or minimum ages to get certified) operating a motorized pleasure craft (this includes any watercraft with a motor, be it a sailboat fitted with an auxiliary motor, or even an electric motor on a canoe) need to hold a Pleasure Craft Operator Card. The purpose of the exam is to ensure that all people operating powered boats are familiar with national safety standards. It is mandatory to carry this card on your person if you are operating a powered boat. There are fines for operating vessels when impaired by alcohol or drugs.

Always wear a personal floatation device when canoeing.

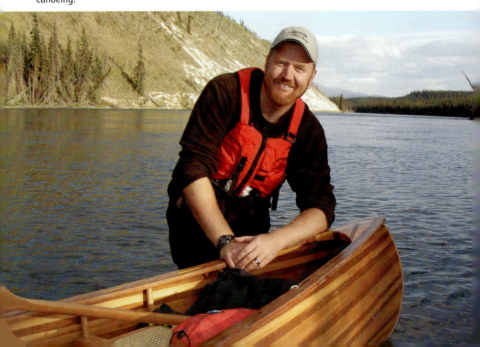

In the interests of safety, there must be personal "life-saving appliances" for all people in the vessel: a lifejacket or Personal Floatation Device (PFD). A Canadian approved "standard lifejacket" (when worn properly) is designed to turn an unconscious person from face down to face up in the water, allowing them to breathe. PFDs are available in a wide range of approved types, sizes and colours. While PFDs are more comfortable than lifejackets because they are designed for constant wear, they do not generally offer the same level of protection as life jackets.

The course provides key information regarding boating accidents, including what to do if a boat capsizes or is swamped with water and how to deal with other emergencies such as fire. Immersion in cold water kills, so there is a section on how to treat victims of immersion and hypothermia. In short, this is an excellent course for anyone who operates a motor-powered boat.

I've spent a lot of time on the water and will share some of my personal experiences on how to stay safe in canoes, outboard motorboats, jet boats, etc.

Before you head out, double check to see that all the mandatory safety equipment as required by Transport Canada, which varies depending on the type and size of the watercraft, is on board.

If you don't know how to swim, you probably shouldn't be on the water because there's always a danger of going overboard, no matter how experienced you might be. **You should take swimming lessons, so you don't endanger your safety or those of members in your party. Transport Canada advises that almost 90 percent of the 180 Canadians (on average) who die in boating incidents every year were not properly wearing a lifejacket or PFD. Nearly 70 percent capsized or fell overboard from a small open boat.** If there's any amount of chop on a lake, be sure to wear your life jacket, and regardless of the weather,

> **If you don't know how to swim, you probably shouldn't be on the water because there's always a danger of going overboard, no matter how experienced you might be.**

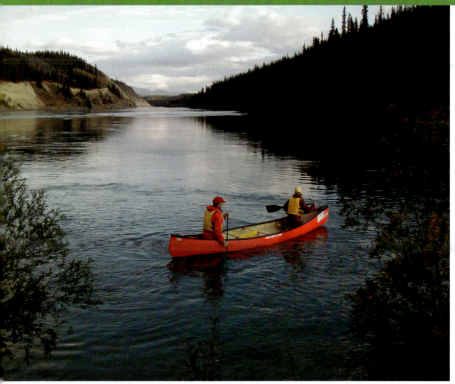

Never stand up in a canoe; it is dangerous.

always wear a life jacket in a canoe, which can capsize even in calm water if there's any degree of imbalance. Never stand up in a canoe, unless it is a "freighter" canoe, which are stable. **The single most important thing that one can do to prevent drowning is to always wear a properly adjusted PFD or lifejacket of appropriate type, size and fit when on the water.**

Transport Canada requires that paddlers carry certain safety items on canoes, kayaks and even kiteboards and stand-up paddleboards. The minimum you need is a PFD and sound signaling device, beyond that, the required equipment varies by type and length of your boat and where and when you plan to paddle. The "International Rating System" classifies rapids as follows:

- **Class A** - Lake water. Still. No perceptible movement.
- **Class I** - Easy. Smooth water; light riffles; clear passages, occasional sand banks and gentle curves. The most difficult problems might arise when paddling around bridges and other obvious obstructions.
- **Class II** - Moderate. Medium-quick water; rapids with regular waves; clear and open passages between rocks and ledges. Maneuvering required. Best handled by intermediates who can maneuver canoes and read water.

- **Class III** - Moderately difficult. Numerous high and irregular waves; rocks and eddies with passages clear but narrow and requiring experience to run. Visual inspection required if rapids are unknown. Open canoes without flotation bags will have difficulty. These rapids are best left to canoeists with expert skills.

- **Class IV** - Difficult. Long and powerful rapids and standing waves; souse holes and boiling eddies. Powerful and precise maneuvering required. Visual inspection mandatory. Cannot be run in canoes unless the craft is decked or properly equipped with flotation bags. Advance preparations for possible rescue work important.

- **Class V** - Extremely difficult. Long and violent rapids that follow each other almost without interruption. River filled with obstructions. Big drops and violent currents. Extremely steep gradient. Even reconnoitering may be difficult. Rescue preparations mandatory. Can be run only by top experts in specially equipped whitewater canoes, decked craft, and kayaks.

- **Class VI** - Extraordinarily difficult. Paddlers face constant threat of death because of extreme danger. Navigable only when water levels and conditions are favorable. This violent whitewater should be left to paddlers of Olympic ability. Every safety precaution must be taken.

By law, all Canadians must have a Pleasure Craft Operator Card to operate powered boats.

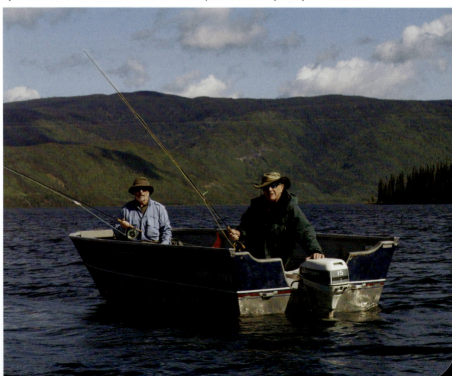

Outboard Motorboats and Electric Motors

If you're boating in an outboard motorboat, check to see that the bung plug is firmly in place. There are always incidents where boats take on water because the bung plug is missing or comes loose. This is where a bailing device is imperative to drain the water.

If there is any chance at all that the gasoline supply might be contaminated with water, be sure to filter it with a chamois when filling the gasoline tank. Otherwise, the motor will stall and be hard to restart, which could spell trouble in some circumstance.

Be extra cautious when boating in shallow water in lakes and rivers, so you don't damage the propeller. Older models of outboard motors had a shear pin in the propeller that would fracture if the propeller hit a hard object. The propeller would be immobilized so as to minimize damage. Using some pliers,

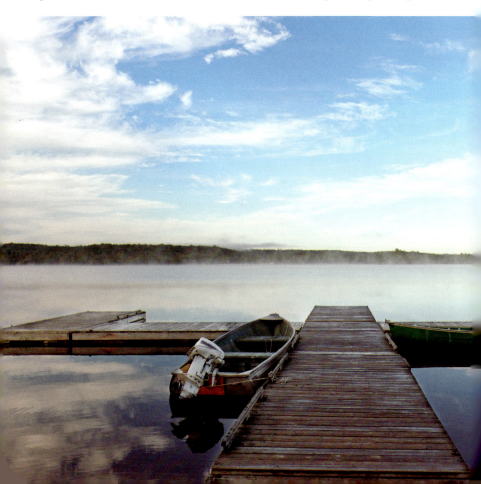

you could remove the cotter pin that held the propeller to the shaft of the motor, replace the pin and you'd be back in business. On modern outboard motors, the propellers have a fracture plane so part of the propeller breaks off before any major damage is done to a shaft and the propeller might have to be scrapped. You should always carry a spare propeller and the tools necessary to repair or replace it if necessary.

If you're using an electric motor on a freighter canoe or cartop boat, it is a good idea to carry extra batteries, especially if it's cold outside, and even a spare electric motor if you're in a remote location, as a backup. An onboard battery charger can also be a life saver. A freighter canoe is difficult to paddle, while a cartop boat can be paddled with oars, and both boats are very hard to steer without power.

My personal experience while boating on lakes is this: if I see whitecaps, danger lurks for pleasure craft, and if the wind is whipping water off the top of whitecaps, you should stay on shore until winds calm down. The trough between waves can be several metres in depth during a storm and this can carry over with huge swells for hours afterwards.

Major rivers in northern Canada can be very intimidating, many of which are fraught with treacherous back eddies, chutes, drift piles, rapids, sweepers, whirlpools, and waterfalls. They're huge, more than mile across, swift and turbulent and often heavily laden with silt. Travel on Canada's large rivers during the spring can be perilous, following ice breakup during the runoff when huge sections of treed banks can give way and wash into the river. With all the debris in the water, navigation can be extremely hazardous.

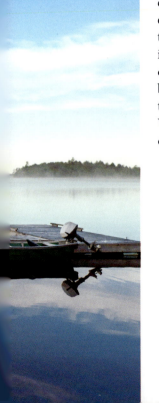

Major rivers in northern Canada can be very intimidating, many of which are fraught with treacherous back eddies, chutes, drift piles, rapids, sweepers, whirlpools, and waterfalls.

Off-highway Vehicle Travel

I've had the good fortune to have travelled on snowmobiles, all-terrain vehicles (i.e., ATV's, popularly called off-highway vehicles or quads) and dirt bikes into backcountry areas I would have never been able to visit otherwise. While I normally prefer hiking over riding these types of vehicles, I can certainly understand their appeal because they really are exciting to ride.

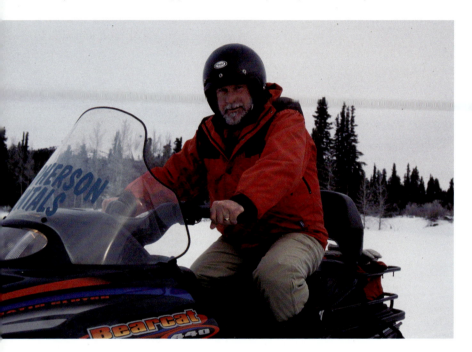

Snowmobiles

Without question, some of the most exciting outdoor adventures I've ever made have been on snowmobiles in the Alberta Rockies and rugged mountain ranges in the Yukon near Dawson City and Whitehorse. In fact, perhaps the greatest backcountry adventure I've ever experienced was orchestrated for me by a local snowmobile association in Pincher Creek, Alberta.

Snowmobile Apparel, Hazards and Travel Guidelines

It is imperative to be properly dressed when snowmobiling in Canada. Snow suits that are windproof and insulated against the cold, insulated boots and gloves are essential, and a helmet is mandatory.

Travel Guidelines

1. Always travel with a buddy[s].
2. Tell other people where you are going and when you are expected back.
3. Bring an extra set of warm clothing and consider purchasing a floatation snowmobile suit.
4. Spread out the weight of snow machines [when travelling across ice] and do not park them close together on the ice.

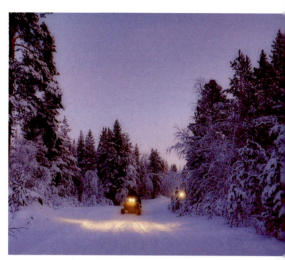

5. Ensure you have the following safety equipment with you: ice picks, rope, cellphone packed in a waterproof container, first aid kit, flashlight, waterproof matches or lighter, tool kit, candles and survival blanket.
6. As when using the road system, do not drive a snow machine while under the influence of drugs and/or alcohol.

The City of Yellowknife recommends "When walking on the ice 'light up'. Wear reflective clothing and/or a form of illumination to ensure snow machine operators can see you. Be aware of your surroundings."

7. Keep the snowmobile in good working order, and do a pre-ride inspection before every trip.
8. Wear a proper-fitting safety-certified snowmobile helmet and make sure to have it buckled up at all times. The chinstrap should be snug.
9. Wear a wind-resistant and water-repellent snowmobile suit or a buoyant snowmobile suit if you travel over frozen water.
10. Dress in layers to maintain proper body warmth and prevent hands and feet from freezing.
11. Wear a turtleneck sweater or neck warmer instead of a scarf that can catch in moving parts.
12. Wear reflective clothing when riding.
13. Carry a first-aid kit, an emergency tool kit, an extra key, and a survival kit that includes flares. Carry a cellular phone if you're in an area with service.
14. Carry an avalanche beacon, probe and shovel, and make sure everyone knows how to use them in the event of an avalanche in backcountry or mountainous terrain.

Some members of their executive took me on an exhilarating trip in the headwaters of the South Castle River, along the High Rock Range of the Alberta Rockies and into British Columbia. We departed from Beaver Mines Lake and travelled southwards along an unmaintained logging road beside the South Castle River to Scarpe Creek, up the valley and over the summit into Sage Creek (located in British Columbia) before returning to Alberta in Font Creek and then back to the trailhead. This trip took place back in the 1980s in late March, following a dump of about a foot of fresh powder snow. Being in the bush with these locals, who were very experienced snowmobilers, taught me that this was no place for amateurs, and that only experts should venture forth and only in teams in such remote mountainous areas.

One of the members of the snowmobile club had a small motors business, and he was kept busy during the trip repairing machines that broke down. A day earlier, we had to tow one machine back to the trailhead because he wasn't able to repair it. The leaders of the local snowmobile club all had high performance snow machines with high altitude carburetor jets and special paddles on their snow machine tracks for added traction in deep, powder snow. They were equipped with avalanche beacons and survival gear. Plus, they had customized chains to fit over the front skis on the snowmobiles to slow their descent off mountains. (A couple of years following my hair-raising adventure two of the club members died in an avalanche—despite being fully prepared for emergencies—in the same area which receives record amount of snow each year.)

About 20 feet of snow falls in the area annually in the headwaters of the Castle River, a lot of it in late winter, and avalanches are not uncommon. I don't think that my heart stopped thumping during the entire, frightening trip. I don't recall how many time members of the entourage got stuck but doing so was routine. A snowmobile weighs about 450 pounds and requires some grit and savvy, and sometimes a shovel to clear a path forward, to get it going again after it gets stuck.

Don't try these kinds of trips unless you're in good shape and are relatively strong, because you'll be on your own for much of the time. One of the members crashed his machine into another snowmobile when he couldn't find the kill switch. He ended up with quite a gash in his nose that took some time to stop the bleeding. We had to snowmobile over top of the Continental Divide into British Columbia before we could make it to a mountain pass that would take us back into Alberta, where were chained up the skis to slow our descent. It was impossible to slow the heavy machines very much, and there were some wrecks with a few machines crashing into trees and free-falling off cliffs.

It was also impossible for members of the group to stay together. At times, it was everyman for himself. When we finally re-grouped in Font Creek and made our way back to Beaver Mines Lake, I thanked my lucky stars.

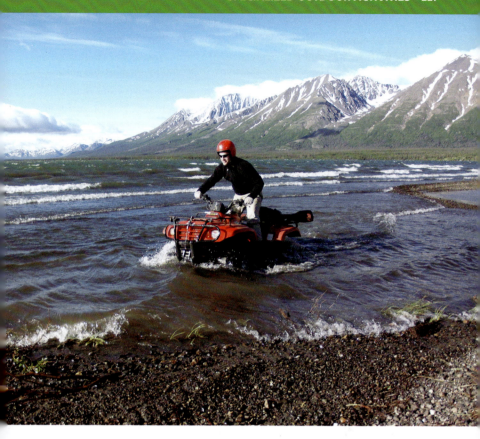

All-terrain Vehicles (ATVs) and Dirt Bikes

The most popular all-terrain vehicles (ATVs) in Canada are quads, and they come in many models that feature different shapes and sizes. Dirt bikes also fall into the ATV category. While you might wonder what they have to do with outdoor survival, you can get into a whole lot of trouble if you don't know how to operate them in the backcountry. Quads and dirt bikes are heavy, powerful machines, and they should not be used by children. Take an ATV operator training course from a trained instructor. The Canada Safety Council offers ATV rider courses that include training on using controls, riding terrain, turning and climbing hills. Adults should only operate them after having received some instruction on their operating features along with some practice. If they roll over or skid you could suffer serious and even fatal harm. Quads are notorious for getting stuck in mudholes, so you must be equipped to get them unstuck or risk having to spend time in the bush until you might be rescued. On dirt bikes, protective clothing is recommended in case of mishaps to protect your body from road rash in the case of falls. Safety helmets should be worn at all times.

By way of example, Alberta Health statistics outline just how serious mishaps with ATVs can be, and these records are probably representative of Canada as a whole: Between 2010 and 2014, 85 Albertans died while riding ATVs. Of those 85, 17 were 16 years and younger. Because more males ride ATVs, more males are injured or killed than females. Head injuries are a major cause of ATV related deaths at 40%. The following common-sense operating guidelines are recommended by Alberta Health:

1. Looking first means thinking ahead. You do this by learning about and understanding the risks and making a plan to manage them.
2. Keep your ATV in good repair. Make sure it has a working headlight, tail light, and muffler.
3. Ride during daylight hours and on flat or gently sloping terrain.
4. Respect the rights of others on the trails (like hikers, cyclists, horseback riders, and animals).
5. Know what the possible hazards are in your riding area. If you don't know the area, find someone who does and ride with them the first few trips.
6. Obey posted signs and stay on the trails. Going off marked trails can mean coming face to face with the unexpected—like ditches, drop offs, cliffs, or trees.
7. Know the local weather conditions. Weather affects the trails.

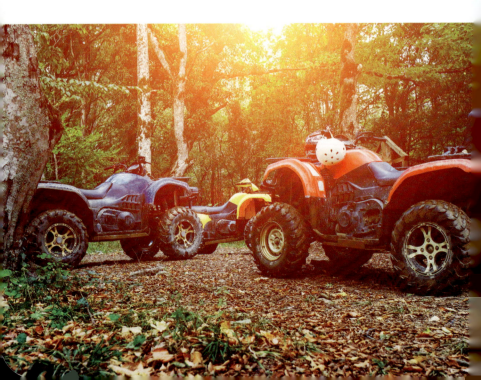

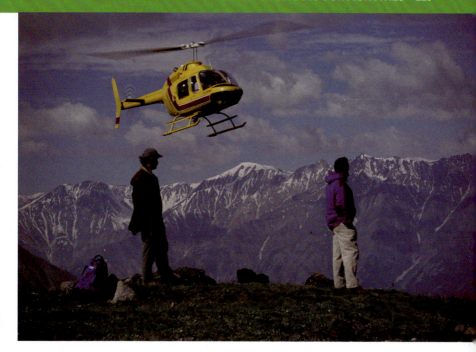

Helicopter and Plane Crashes, Contingencies

I believe that most people think they will never experience a plane or helicopter crash, and they are probably right. However, I also believe that folks who do a lot of flying are naïve if they think they won't crash at some point, because the odds are good that something will eventually go wrong. There are various common reasons for crashes, such as bad weather, mechanical breakdowns and pilot error. I've done a lot of flying around the world and in all parts of Canada on commercial airlines, bush planes and helicopters, so I speak from experience. I am going to describe a few events that have happened to me personally to illustrate the role that mechanical breakdowns, pilot error and weather can play in these events and the importance of being prepared for a crash. Things happen very quickly during crashes. Often, there's no time to transmit a "Mayday" call, and it can turn out to be every man for themselves.

> **There are various common reasons for crashes, such as bad weather, mechanical breakdowns and pilot error.**

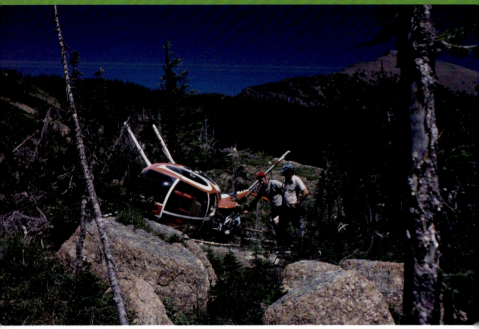

Bighorn Helicopters Hughes 500 crash

Helicopters

The most frightening and terrifying crash I've experienced happened on Tuesday, July 25, 1978, in southwestern Alberta's Rocky Mountains. I was on a job with the Alberta government, at the time surveying some alpine lakes on Three Lakes Ridge, which is on the High Rock Range south of the popular Castle Mountain Resort in the headwaters of the West Castle River. I had contracted a helicopter from Bighorn Helicopters in Fernie, British Columbia that was piloted by Jim Drozduk. He was a veteran pilot whose aviation skills likely saved my life and that of my co-worker, Lorne Fitch. Piloting one of these machines requires great skill and dexterity. Drozduk was flying a Hughes 500 helicopter, a reliable workhorse machine that is highly maneuverable (these choppers date back to the war in Vietnam). I'd flown with Drozduk many times and trusted his judgement in the Alberta mountains, where flying conditions can sometimes be hazardous. Before each and every flight, I would always tell charter pilots not to take any chances if they judge flying conditions to be dangerous, because I didn't want any accidents. I say this because charter pilots get paid by the hour; they're not on salary, so some will take chances to please a client.

After Fitch and I had completed a survey of one of the lakes on Three Lakes Ridge, we packed up our sampling gear and loaded it back into the chopper to get ready to work on one of the other nearby lakes.

The pilot, Drozduk, went through all of the normal takeoff procedures, and the Hughes 500 slowly became airborne. The winds were calm. He nosed the chopper toward the mountain downslope as he gained about 50 feet in elevation. Fitch was sitting in the cockpit to the right of Drozduk. I was strapped into a seat in the rear seating area, behind Fitch. As Drozduk took off, I knew something was wrong. The motor didn't have the normal pitch. I could sense that it was being starved of fuel required for flight. Before it reached cruising altitude it started to lose altitude, and Drozduk nosed the machine down, toward the valley we had ascended earlier that morning. As we flew into the area, I carefully studied the lay of the land in case we would need to walk out, because I'd never been in the area before and wasn't familiar with the terrain. In a later conversation, the pilot told me he'd done the same thing and noted an old seismic line in the valley bottom. Directly ahead was an old burn where a forest fire had gone through a lodgepole pine forest many years ago. Most of the trees were still standing, their trunks scarred by fire. The burn was huge, maybe half a mile in length. I didn't know this at the time, but Drozduk had turned the chopper towards the seismic line below the burn, in the valley bottom, because he felt he could land there, in a pinch. No other openings were in sight.

Pilots are trained to land a helicopter by autorotation if there's an engine failure. Drozduk told me that he practiced this maneuver during flights between Calgary (where the machine was routinely serviced) and his base in Fernie. Under the circumstances, it was impossible to autorotate straight down because of the pitch in the valley. We were going to crash land, period. As the machine continued to lose altitude, it started to mow down trunks of the burned pine trees and what was left of their branches. The sound was terrifying as the rotor blades of the helicopter cut

Helicopter pilots go through the following process prior to takeoff, into the wind:

1. First, the pilot opens the throttle completely to increase the speed of the rotor.

2. Next, he or she pulls up slowly on the collective. The collective control raises the entire swash plate assembly as a unit. This has the effect of changing the pitch of all rotor blades by the same amount simultaneously.

3. As the pilot increases collective pitch, he or she depresses the left foot pedal to counteract the torque produced by the main rotor.

4. The pilot keeps pulling up slowly on the collective while depressing the left foot pedal.

5. When the amount of lift being produced by the rotor exceeds the weight of the helicopter, the aircraft will get light on its skids and slowly leave the ground.

6. At this point, the pilot feels the cyclic become sensitive. He or she grips the cyclic and, in most cases, nudges the helicopter forward [just prior to actual takeoff].

After you've flown in a helicopter as many times as I have, you know what to listen for and how the various sounds of the engine and rotors signal a normal takeoff.

through the tree trunks, made worse as the fuselage and skids plowed into them head on. I stopped breathing, wondering how much pounding the chopper could take before it broke apart or the pilot was impaled by a tree. I tightened my seat belt and prayed for the best. After what seemed like forever, we cleared the burn. Finally, the chopper hit the rocky ground, on a steep slope, and skidded into a boulder, a glacial erratic the size of a Volkswagen. As it did so the chopper flipped over, more or less on its back. We were basically upside down for a while, the rotor blades still turning and smashing against the massive boulder. I could smell jet fuel in the cockpit. The roaring sound was absolutely deafening. I undid my seat belt and braced my feet against the partition separating the rear seating area from the cockpit. Thoughts of fire and being burned alive raced through my mind. Amid the cacophony of the roaring engine and the rotor blades being torn apart I could see Drozduk being thrown wildly around in his seat. His head was down, and I thought he might be dead as he gyrated in his seat. I couldn't see Fitch. I had no idea if he was dead or alive. My thoughts were on escape. However, I didn't dare try to exit the helicopter for fear of being killed by the rotating rotor blades. Finally, the motor stopped running, and the rotor blades no longer smashed against the car-sized boulder. Frantically, I opened the back door and pulled myself out, a bit dazed but mobile. After I hit the ground, I took several steps away from the chopper taking in the scene. I looked around for signs of fire; seeing none, I climbed back on the machine. I opened the front door, not knowing what I'd find. Fortunately, it looked like both Fitch and Drozduk were okay. I helped them out and we retreated from the scene to take stock of the situation. My heart was still pounding. I'd never felt such a massive buildup of body heat before, especially in my chest. I had an overwhelming thirst. Seeing that there was no imminent danger, Drozduk retrieved a fire extinguisher from the downed helicopter and sprayed down the machine, as a precaution. It may sound hard to believe, but we all escaped the crash without so much as a scratch.

    The chopper was later air lifted out of the crash site and examined by Transport Canada officials. As it turned out, there was a problem with the fuel injector that was not feeding enough jet fuel to the engine. While Drozduk was being thrown around the fuselage he was doing what he was trained to do, although I didn't know it until afterwards. He was trying to shut off the engine. First, he turned the key off. Nothing happened. Next, he turned the fuel line off. Again, nothing happened. Finally, he turned off the battery switch, which shut off the engine.

I always made it a point to wear suitable hiking boots with Vibram soles so I could kick a door off a helicopter if necessary. While I didn't have to kick my way out of the downed machine this time, the boots paid off, because we had to hike about 15 km before we encountered an Alberta Forest Service vehicle in the area and hitched a ride back to Blairmore, Alberta. This experience changed my life forever. It made me ever grateful for what I have and all the joys of life that folks tend to take for granted.

The next year, while flying in a charter Jet Ranger helicopter along the Livingstone Range in southwestern Alberta, we got caught up in fierce Chinook winds that were so strong the pilot could only fly forward; he couldn't turn the machine around to get out of the wind. The downdrafts were so strong, they plunged the chopper hundreds of feet, almost to ground, before the pilot could regain altitude. He told me later that he'd never experienced such strong winds, and we were lucky we didn't crash.

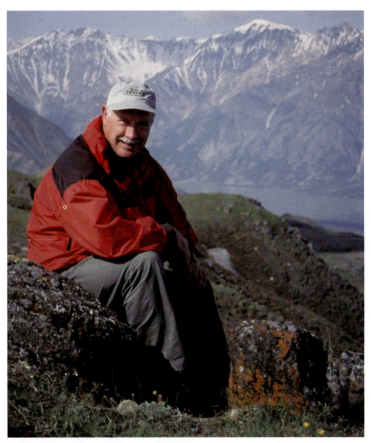

Author, Outpost Mountain, Yukon heli-hiking

Bush Planes

In 1966, I was flying with a bush pilot who was ferrying in supplies to survey Wylie Lake north of Lake Athabasca in northeastern Alberta. He was flying a Cessna 172 float plane, loaded to capacity. We circled the lake in search of a suitable campsite with a sandy beach. Sandy beaches are ideal for landing, because there is little danger of damaging the floats. Besides, it is easier to load and unload cargo than on more rugged beaches. We were also hoping to find a campsite strategically located near the epicentre of the lake to make the survey go faster. The pilot decided on a wide, sandy beach that was bordered by a forest of black spruce and jack pine.

Planes land into the wind and take off into the wind. Pilots try to avoid cross winds, because they can push a plane sideways and cause problems while landing or taking off. There was a wind from the northwest on this day, which is the prevailing wind direction in the area. There were waves on the water that the pilot wanted to avoid as much as possible, so he cut the landing short. The problem was that he misjudged how much water he needed to land safely.

As soon as he touched down, I knew we were in trouble. The landing speed on a Cessna 172 is about 55-65 knots (63-75 mph) depending on the payload, with flaps down. Some float planes, though, have a history of leaky floats. If they had taken on water, the plane would weigh more, which would complicate

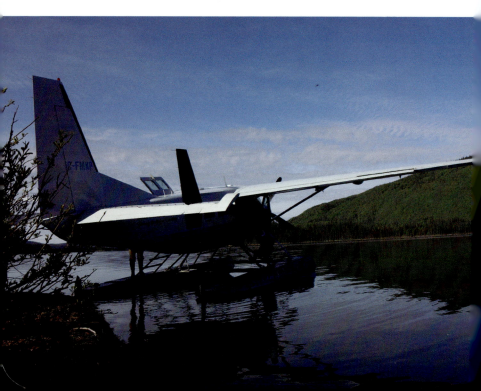

matters. Regardless, most pilots will land well out into a lake and take some extra time to taxi to shore. This one didn't, and we ended up landing short with the plane speeding quickly toward the beach. The pilot told me to brace myself and hang on for a hard landing on shore. The trees were coming up fast, and my hope was that we wouldn't go too far up the sandy beach and wreck the plane and/or injure ourselves.

When the plane finally came to a stop, it was well beached to say the least. However, after we unloaded it, we managed to wiggle it back into the lake to fly again. However, this was a close call and could have easily had a worse ending.

On another occasion, my son, Myles, and I were flying on a charter flight from the Tree River to Kugluktuk, Nunavut (a remote Inuit community) in a de Havilland Canada DHC-3 *Otter,* which is one of the best bush planes ever built, up there with the legendary de Havilland DHC-2 Beaver. Both of these planes are single-engine, high-wing propeller-driven short takeoff and landing (STOL) aircraft developed and manufactured by de Havilland Canada. I was to find out later that the pilot of the Otter had never landed in the Arctic Ocean at Kugluktuk. The Otter was loaded to near capacity with passengers and their gear. Flying conditions were ideal. Everyone was strapped into their seats, as is mandatory by law. The pilot's flight course was a straight shot from the Tree River west to Kugluktuk at a cruising speed of about 120 mph over a distance of 136 km. Veteran bush pilot Larry Nagy said in an email, "When doing your final approach, you religiously maintain 80 mph...full flaps, flare around 60-65 mph depending on [the Otter's] load."

The pilot touched down on the Arctic Ocean, which was fairly smooth, but at low tide. The float plane sped toward the Inuit settlement of Kugluktuk. Without warning, it came to a sudden stop and I mean sudden, as it plowed into a submerged sandbar out in the ocean. Rats! Passengers would have crashed into the wall if they hadn't been wearing seat belts, and the cargo would have done likewise if it hadn't been strapped down. We were royally stuck. There was no getting unstuck until the tide came in and the plane floated off the sandbar. Chalk this up to pilot error. If he'd been familiar with the bay, he would have landed closer to Kugluktuk and missed the sandbar, which was apparently well-known by locals. Myles and I had a commercial flight to catch back home to Edmonton so it was with much gratitude that we accepted a boat ride to shore with a local Inuk man, otherwise we would have had to stay over a weekend, and there's precious little accommodation in Kugluktuk.

Contingencies

In one of the most recent Canadian aviation disasters on July 15, 2019, seven men, including the pilot, who were on board an Air Saguenay-owned de Havilland DHC-2 Beaver, perished when it crashed into Mistastin Lake, about 100 km southwest of Nain in Labrador. The cause of the crash remains unknown, and the plane's fuselage was never located. If a float plane crashes on a lake and flips over, it can be very difficult for the passengers to exit the plane. Seconds count and passengers and pilots may not be able to get out of a damaged plane. That is why you should always study the interior of a plane before take-off and note where the exits are located in the event of an emergency.

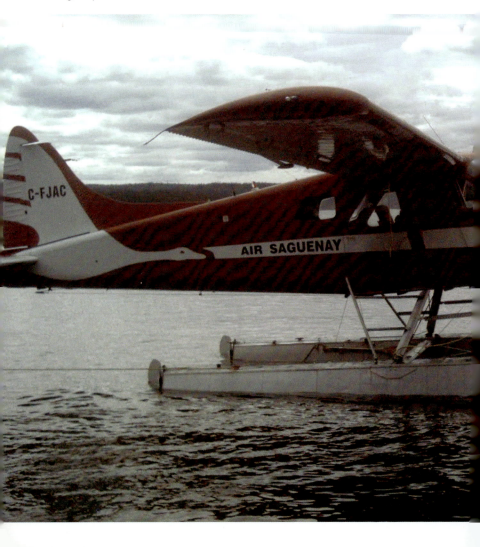

In my experience, bush plane and helicopter pilots are skilled flyers and very safety conscious. They do not take unnecessary risks, but they do fly in remote areas where weather conditions are not always ideal. They always explain safety features before takeoff, where first aid kits, floatation devices and emergency locator beacons (transponders) are located and how to use them. There are strict laws regarding cargo on float planes and all items are weighed before takeoff. It is mandatory to wear seat belts. Pilots will explain what to do in the event of a crash. They will tell you to close helicopter doors carefully, while doors on most bush planes can be slammed shut. You may notice that some pilots wear non-flammable jump suits, hiking boots and crash helmets.

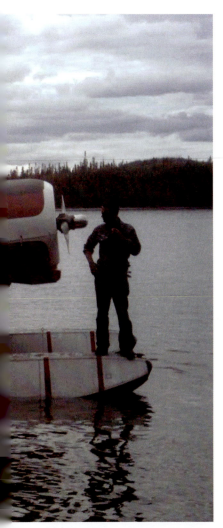

I make it a point not to wear flammable clothing in bush planes and helicopters. Furthermore, I wear boots suitable for hiking, just in case a plane crashes and I have to walk out to civilization. I carry a survival kit on my person (see Survival Kit p. xx for details). I pay attention to the landscape during the flight, noting key landmarks along the way. If possible, I will sit near the tail in planes, because most survivors of plane crashes have been seated in this part of the airplane. I double check the exits and study the nature of the door handles—where they're located on the doors and how they work.

Air Saguenay-owned de Havilland DHC-2 Beaver

Mountain Climbing

In 2020, Parks Canada brought in new rules for climbers on Canada's highest peak, Mount Logan, Yukon after having to rescue eight people in seven years. The new rules include a ban on solo climbing and a moratorium on winter mountaineering in Kluane National Park, Yukon. The moratorium on winter travel runs from November 15 to March 15. Further, climbers are now required to have insurance to cover search and rescue costs for any trip in this national park Icefield's Ranges before they will be issued a climbing permit. Climbers who want to do an expedition in the Icefield Ranges from late March to mid-November require a permit from Parks Canada.

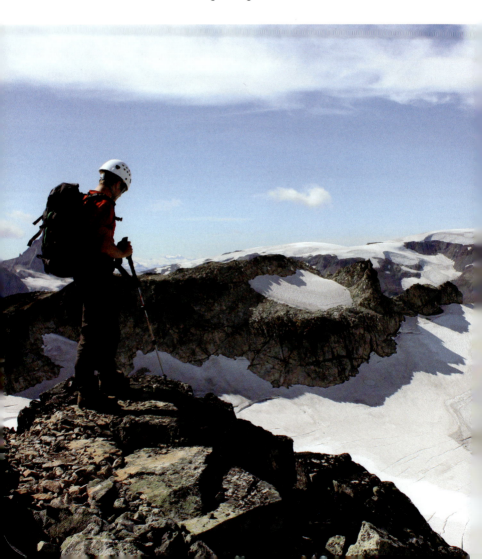

Insurance requirement: Prior to being issued a Mountaineering Permit, climbers must provide proof of insurance, that: "Covers the cost of organized rescue/extraction from the Icefield Ranges for the activities outlined in their permit application to a minimum of CAN $100,000." Climbers requiring rescue will be billed directly for costs associated with extraction. They may then recover these expenses from their insurance provider.

In other Canadian national parks, a backcountry permit is mandatory for anyone planning an overnight trip into the backcountry. The permit is for your own safety. Mountaineers require a backcountry permit to bivouac and may do so in non-vegetated areas only. Alternatively, the Alpine Club of Canada (403-678-3200) operates several mountaineering huts in some parks, such as Banff National Park, that are ideally located for mountaineers.

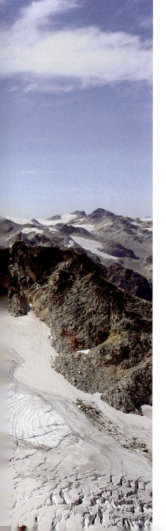

Mountain climbing is not recommended for amateurs, because it is a dangerous and high-risk activity. Only those outdoorspeople with proper training and gear should attempt to climb mountains, because the risk of falls is high. Further, those who climb mountains or hike in Canada's mountainous backcountry should be aware of the importance of acclimation to high altitudes. It takes a person's body a few days to build up red blood corpuscles to carry additional oxygen in the blood, and until this occurs, they will feel fatigued and tired. The Government of Canada cautions that "as altitude increases, the total barometric pressure and partial pressure of oxygen decrease, resulting in hypoxia, which may be associated with decreased exercise performance, increased ventilation and symptoms of lightheadedness, fatigue, altered perceptions and sleep disorders. Although the risk increases with altitude, some susceptible individuals may experience symptoms of altitude-related illness beginning as low as 2500 m (8200 ft)." Elevations around 2500 m are not uncommon in Canada's mountainous areas. Mount Logan, Yukon is Canada's highest peak at 5959 m (19,550 ft.)

Brandywine Mountain in the Coast Mountains of British Columbia

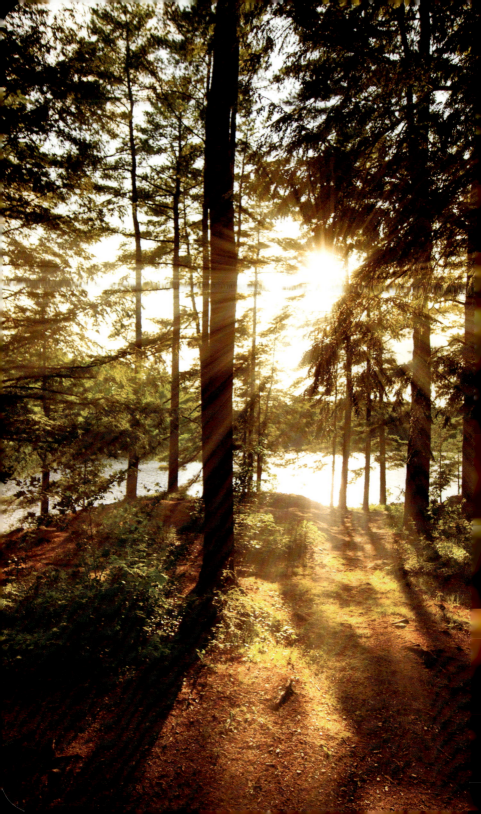

SECTION 4
Reflection

I make a point of reflecting on each day in the outdoors with my companions at day's end. What did we enjoy? Were there any particular highlights? Did anything go wrong? Why? What should we do differently next time around? I also think about these matters if I'm alone.

I carry a notebook to make notes during the day, so I don't forget important details. As an author, I can refer to them later so any works I might write are accurate. I summarize any issues or concerns in a spreadsheet when I return home, following the trip, so I can refer to these notes before taking similar trips in the future. I don't rely on my memory; I don't want to forget important details.

Discussing the next day's plans with your companions is also an important part of the evening conversation. It's best done in a team environment with the goal of reaching a consensus among all members of the party on what you're going to do the next day. Furthermore, it's important to have a positive outlook going forward so that you can build some enthusiasm to surmount any challenges. Don't travel with people who are negative, because they will detract from the important aspects of being outdoors. Negativity in the outdoors will create friction among team members and lead to problems.

I'm a firm believer in planning and organizing trips well ahead of schedule so that all gear is in working order and nothing important is forgotten. There's no substitute for a check list.

Further, there's an old saying that "A good farmer always cleans his tools after a day's work." In the evening,

I make it a point to check my gear, fix anything that's broken and try to get ready for the next day so I have the peace of mind that everything is in working order before I go to sleep. I'll lay out my gear, so everything is organized, including a change of clothes when appropriate. I like to control things that are within my power to control by being prepared should things go wrong to avoid a disaster. I find that I can make my often make my own karma and keep my spirits up by having some good things to look forward to.

Every day in Canada's outdoors is a good day. You will be refreshed having been close to nature. Physical exercise will clear your mind and invigorate your body. You are, however, responsible for your own safety in Canada's outdoors. Remember, cell phone coverage is unreliable, there will be no electricity. Be prepared for extreme weather, predators and trail hazards. If you follow the advice and information in this book, you should have a safe trip with no incidents, and you should be able to enjoy the wonders of Canada's backcountry without any worries.

There is probably no place on earth like Canada that features such great geographic diversity, abundant wildlife and natural wonders. I speak from experience, because I've travelled all the world's continents, except Antarctica. The key is to be prepared for your adventure, make plans that are realistic, network with friends and family so they know where you're going and when you expect to complete your trip, along with what to do as a fallback if something goes wrong.

I've been on outdoor adventures all across Canada, from coast to coast to coast. Some of them have been very challenging and exciting, but that's part of the adventure. I've never felt that I was at risk and made sure that if a problem did develop, I was fully prepared to address it without minimal worries. That's what it's all about, being prepared

To paraphrase Orville Caddy, my Labrador fishing guide, plan for the worst but hope for the best!

Every day in Canada's outdoors is a good day. You will be refreshed having been close to nature. Physical exercise will clear your mind and invigorate your body.

Notes

Notes

Notes

Notes

Notes

Appendix

10 Techniques for catching fish in a survival situation
https://www.outdoorlife.com/blogs/survivalist/10-techniques-catching-fish-survival-situation/

Aerial flares
https://www.orionsignals.com/?s=Aerial+flares

Bear attack PAGE NO LONGER UP
https://calgaryherald.com/news/local-news/bear-involved-in-sundre-attack-was-a-grizzly officials-say/

Crashed float plane in Labrador
https://www.canadianunderwriter.ca/insurance/search-ends-for-crashed-float-plane-in-labrador-1004167081/

Dark water
http://www.alaskaforreal.com/blog/dark-water

Firefly Pro Solas emergency strobe light
https://www.acrartex.com/products/firefly-pro-solas

Get into trouble outdoors — Who pays for the rescue?
http://content.time.com/time/nation/article/0,8599,1892621,00.html

Helicopters
https://science.howstuffworks.com/transport/flight/modern/helicopter7.htm

Appendix

High altitude illnesses
https://www.canada.ca/en/public-health/services/reports-publications/canada-communicable-disease-report-ccdr/monthly-issue/2007-33/statement-on-high-altitude-illnesses.html

Snowmobile safety
There are also several other snowmobile safety tips to keep in mind when in the Canadian outdoors, posted online by the Alberta government. https://www.transportation.alberta.ca/3278.htm).

Snowshoe selection guide
https://lureofthenorth.com/info-hub/snowshoe-selection-guide/

The real reason your parka has a fur trim
https://www.mensjournal.com/style/the-real-reason-your-parka-has-a-fur-trim/

Topographic maps
https://www.nrcan.gc.ca/maps-tools-publications/maps/topographic-maps/10995

Trail ride vacations
http://trailridevacations.com/)

What is survival rule of fours
https://www.thesmartsurvivalist.com/what-is-survival-rule-of-fours/

Index

A

ABCDE rule, see *Triage*
Accelerants, see *Fire*
Alberta, 18, 36, 55, 122, 124, 136, 157, 160, 161, 176, 187, 188, 190, 197, 198, 201, 202, 214, 228
All-terrain vehicles (ATV), 224, 227
Animal snares, 133
Animal tracks, 114, 182
Animal traps 131, 133
   Deadfall trap, 134
   Rabbit snare, 133
Asparagus, see *Edible plants*
Avalanche, 160–163
   Avalanche beacon, 161, 163, 225
   RECCO Avalanche System, 162
Axe, 55, 67–69, 90, 93, 106, 108, 109, 150, 188

B

Backcountry, 15, 19, 34, 38, 55, 81, 83, 115, 120, 152, 153, 160, 161, 175, 215, 224, 225, 227, 239
Backpack, 53, 58, 184
Bear, 17–19, 33, 64, 103, 109, 122, 126, 172, 173, 175–185, 188, 200, 203
   Black bear 19, 103, 126, 175–177, 180–184, 185
   Grizzly bear, 18, 19, 103, 176, 177, 179–181, 183, 184
   Polar bear, 175, 179, 185
Bear attacks, 17, 19, 184, 185
   Predatory attack, 184
   Provoked attack, 184
Bearberries or kinnikinnick, see *Edible plants*
Bird eggs, 129
Bison, 186
Black bear, see *Bear*
Blackberries, raspberries and cloudberry, see *Edible plants*
Bleeding, see *First aid*
Blueberries and huckleberries, see *Edible plants*
Blisters, see *First aid*
Bloodroot, see *Poisonous plants*
Boat safety, 217–223
   Boating Safety Course, 218
   Electric motors, 218, 222
   Motorboats, 218, 222
   Pleasure Craft Operator Card, 218
Bough bed, see *Shelter*
Breaking fast, see *First aid*
British Columbia, 18, 19, 33, 36, 55, 75, 122, 124, 125, 136, 158, 160, 161, 164, 171, 176, 186–188, 190, 192–194, 196–198, 201, 202, 211
Broken bones, see *First aid*
Bug spray, see *Survival kit*
Bush planes, 229, 234, 235, 237

C

Camp stove, see *Food*
Campsite, 55, 102, 103, 159, 173, 181, 198, 200
Canoe (canoeing), 217, 218, 220, 223
Car survival, 214
Cattails, see *Edible plants*
Celestial, see *Navigation*
Chokecherries, see *Edible plants*
Clothing, 34, 39, 48–51, 57, 64, 87, 93, 94, 103, 140, 147, 149, 200, 202, 214, 225, 227, 237
   Gore-Tex, 50, 52
   Hat, 52, 55, 148, 200
   Polar fleece, 50
   Thinsulate, 50, 52
Communication technology, 77–81
   High frequency radio, 77

Index

Low frequency radio, 77
Satellite phone, 79
inReach global satellite technology, 80
Spot X, 81
Compass, see *Navigation*
Concussion, see *First aid*
Contingency plan, 34, 65, 175, 229, 236
Cougar, 33, 103, 109, 175, 187, 188
Coyote, 175, 189
CPR, see *First aid*
Cranberries, see *Edible plants*
Currants, see *Edible plants*
Cuts, see *First aid*

D

Dehydration, see *First aid*
Dirt bikes, 224, 227
Drinking water, 113–114
   Boiling, 117
   Charcoal filter, 118
   Chlorine dioxide tablets, 119
   DIY rock and sand filter, 118
   Giardia, 116
   Iodine tablets, 118
   LifeStraw, 119
   Melting snow, 118
   Potassium permanganate, 119
   Solar still, 115
   Water filtration, 115, 116
   Water purification, 115–119
Drowning, 17, 142, 218, 220

E

Edible plants, 120–126
   Asparagus, 121
   Bearberries or kinnikinnick, 122
   Blackberries, raspberries and cloudberry, 121
   Blueberries and huckleberries, 122
   Cattails, 123
   Chokecherries, 124
   Cranberries, 123
   Currants, 124
   Morels, 125
   Raspberries. 125
   Saskatoon berries, 126
   Strawberries, 126
Elk, 190
Eye injuries, see *First aid*

F

Fallen tree shelter, see *Shelter*
Finding water, 113–115
   Animal tracks and trails, 114
   Digging, 114
   Freshwater springs, 113
   Head downhill, 113
   Ice and snow, 114
   Morning dew, 115
   Rainwater, 114
   Streams and lakes, 115
   Vegetation moisture, 113
Fire, 39, 41, 55, 87, 88, 90, 91, 93, 94, 96–99, 101–104, 105, 107, 108, 114, 118, 125, 132, 147, 169, 199, 212
   Accelerants, 99
      Cotton ball & petroleum jelly, 99
      Dryer lint, 99
      Hand sanitizer & gauze pad, 99
      Wax & fibre, 99
   Firewood, 93
      Hardwood, 91
      Softwood, 91
   Fire location, 93
   Fire pit, 94
   Fire safety, 101
   Fire tending, 101
   Fire triangle, 90

Index

How to start a fire, 94
    Bow drill, 98
    Fire plough, 98
    Hand drill, 98
    Flint & steel method, 97
    Log cabin method, 96
    Magnifying glass method, 97
    Steel wool & battery method, 97
    Teepee method, 96
    Kindling, 90
    Tinder, 90
First aid, 42, 46, 47, 138, 139, 150, 151, 156, 157, 163, 175, 198,
    Bleeding, 46, 150–152, 155
    Blisters, 56, 127, 145
    Breaking fast, 38
    Broken bones, 152, 153
    Concussion, 154, 211
    CPR, 142, 143
    Cuts, 39, 46, 93, 150–152
    Dehydration, 148
    Eye injuries, 155
    Frostbite, 52, 53, 144–146
    Head injuries, 154, 161, 228
    Heat exhaustion, see *Heatstroke*
    Heatstroke, 148
    Hypothermia, 34, 49, 53, 64, 94, 144, 146, 147, 170, 175, 211, 219
    Infection, 46, 55, 150, 151, 157, 199, 201–203
    Insect bites, 157, 200
    Shock, 150, 175
    Snake bites, 156, 157, 198
    Sprain, 138, 152, 153, 165, 211
    Ticks, see *Ticks*
    Wounds, 39, 46, 47, 150–152, 157
First aid kit, 42, 46, 47, 151, 225
    Bug spray, 47
    Commercial first aid kit, 47
    Pocket-size first aid kit, 47
    Sunscreen, 47

Fishing, 39–41, 44, 66, 120, 135–137
    Basket trap, 136
    Dip nets, 135
    DIY fishing hook, 137
    Fish poisons, 136
    Fish spears, 136
    Fishing hook, 41, 66
    Fishing line, 40, 136
    Fishing lure, 41
    Gill nets, 135
    Gorge hook, 136
    Hand fishing, 135
    Hand lines, 136
    Legalities, 137
    Striking irons, 136
Flare, 40, 42, 45, 58, 64, 183, 225
Flashlight, 42, 45, 58, 59, 129, 198, 225
Floods, 164
    Flash floods, 164
    Spring floods, 164
Food
    Camp stove, 101
    Fool hen, 131, 132
    High-energy snacks, 44
    Porcupine, 131
    Rabbit, 133, 134
    Trapping, 120
Fool hen, see *Food*
Footwear, 48, 56, 57, 87
    Vibram, 56, 57, 233
Foraging, 120, 127–130
    Bird eggs, 129
    Insects, 130
    Nuts and seeds, 129
Forester's tent, see *Shelter*
Frostbite, see *First aid*

G

Google Earth, see *Maps*
Gore-Tex, see *Clothing*

Index

GPS, see *Navigation*
Grizzly bear, see *Bears*

H

Hammock, 106
Hatchet, 67, 68, 69, 106, 108, 150
Hat, see *Clothing*
Head injuries, see *First aid*
Headlamp, 58, 59, 161
Heat exhaustion, see *First aid*
Heater, catalytic
Heater, methanol
Heatstroke, see *First aid*
Helicopter, 211, 229–231, 237
High-energy snacks, see *Food*
Hunting, 19, 44, 133, 137
    Legalities, 137
Hypothermia, see *First aid*

I

Ice, 114, 156, 168–170, 215, 223, 225
    Travel on ice, 168–170
Igloo, see *Shelter*
Indigenous, 11, 13, 14, 21, 24, 60, 63, 129, 135
Infection, see *First aid*
Insects, see *Foraging*
    Insect bites, see *First aid*
Inuit, 13, 14, 27, 49, 105, 155, 175, 235

K

Knives, 65, 66, 150
Knots, 207–210
    Bow (bowline) knot, 207
    Half hitch, 208
    Overhand knot, 209
    Slip knot, 210

L

Landslides, 160
Layering, 52
Leaf structure, see *Shelter*
Lean-to shelter, see *Shelter*
Lean-to tent, see *Shelter*
Leather gloves, 55, 93
Leatherman, 46, 65, 66
Lifejacket, 218–220
Lighter, 44, 94, 97, 99, 225
Log cabin method, see *Fire*

M

Magnifying glass method, see *Fire*
Maps, 35, 80–85, 162, 205
    Google Earth, 82, 85
    Topographic maps, 80, 83–85, 205
Matches, 41, 42, 44, 45, 58, 94, 97, 99, 167, 225
Mattress, 74, 76, 109
Merino wool, 56
Métis, 13, 14
Moose, 191, 192
Morels, see *Edible plants*
Mountain climbing, 139, 238, 239
Mountaineer's tent, see *Shelter*
Muskeg, 34, 111, 115, 123, 171

N

Natural shelters and caves, see *Shelter*
Navigation
    Celestial navigation, 206
    Compass, 80, 85, 88, 205
    GPS, 80–82, **206**
Newfoundland & Labrador, 36, 60, 164, 192, 195, 199
Northwest Territories, 47, 128, 176, 186, 192, 195

Index

O
Omni-Heat, 50

P
Personal floatation device (PFD), 169, 218–220
Plane crash, 39, 229, 236, 237
Pocket survival kit, see *Survival kit*
Pocketknife, 40, 65, 66
Poison ivy and poison oak, see *Poisonous plants*
Poisonous plants, 127–128
    Bloodroot, 127
    Poison ivy and poison oak, 127
    Snowberry, 128
    Water-hemlocks, 128
Polar bears, see *Bear*
Polar fleece, see *Clothing*
Porcupines, see *Food*

Q
Quinzee hut, see *Shelter*

R
Rabbit, see *Food*
Rabbit snare, see *Animal snares*
Raingear, 55
Rapids, 83, 85, 220, 221, 223
Raspberries, see *Edible plants*

S
Safety pin, 40
Saskatoon berries, see *Edible plants*
Saws, 67, 69
    Bow saws, 69, 109

Scotch Guard Outdoor Water Shield, 57
Search and rescue (SAR), 20, 87, 120, 199, 211, 238
Shelter
    Bough bed, 107, 109
    Fallen tree shelter, 108
    Forester's tent, 73, 106
    Igloo, 105
    Leaf structure, 108, 109
    Lean-to structure, 106, 107
    Lean-to tent, 73, 106
    Natural shelters and caves, 109
    Quinzee hut, 104
    Snow cave, 105
    Wall tent, 71, 178
Shock, see *First aid*
Signalling, 212, 213
    Smoke signalling, 212
    Whistles, 213
Sleeping bag, 73–75
    Down, 74
    Synthetic, 75
Sleeping pad, see *Mattress*
Slip knot, see *Knots*
Snakes, 109, 156, 157, 195–198
    Snake bites, see *First aid*
    Desert nightsnake, 197
    Massasauga rattlesnake, 196
    Northern pacific rattlesnake, 196
    Prairie (western) rattlesnake, 197, 198
Snake bites, see *First aid*
Snare wire, 39, 40
Snow blindness, 155
Snow cave, see *Shelter*
Snowberry, see *Poisonous plants*
Snowmobile, 160, 163, 168, 170, 224–226

Index

Snowshoes, 60–64
   Algonquin snowshoes, 60
   Bearpaw snowshoes, 63
   Cree snowshoes, 63
   Huron snowshoes, 60
   Ojibwe snowshoes, 63
Solar still, see *Water purification*
Spiders, 201
SPOT X, 81
Sprains, see *First Aid*
Steel wool & battery method, see *Fire*
STOP Method, 88
Strawberries, see *Edible plants*
Sun blindness, 155
Sunglasses, 55, 155, 166
Sunscreen, see *Survival Kit*
Survival kit, 38–42, 47
   Pocket survival kit, 40, 41
   Vehicle survival kit, 42
Survival rule of four, 89
Swimming, 219

T

Tarps, 73, 106, 113
Technology, see *Communication technology*
Teepee method, see *Fire*
Tent, 55, 67, 71–73, 102, 103, 106, 113, 177, 179, 181, 183
Thinsulate, see *Clothing*
Ticks, 202
Tinder, see *Fire*
Topographic, see *Maps*
Transport Canada emergency symbols, 43
Trapping, see *Food*
Trekking poles, 60
Triage, 140

V

Vehicle survival kit, see *Survival kit*
Vibram, see *Footwear*

W

Wall tent, see *Shelter*
Water, see *Finding water*
Water-hemlocks, see *Poisonous plants*
Waterproofing, 57, 71
Weather patterns, 34–37, 42, 48, 158, 159, 239
   Barometric pressure, 158, 159, 239
   Bird behaviour, 158
Whistle, see *Signalling*
Wildlife encounters, 172, 173
Wildlife safety, 175–203
   Bear, see *Bear*
   Bison, see *Bison*
   Cougar, see *Cougar*
   Coyote, see *Coyote*
   Elk, see *Elk*
   Moose, see *Moose*
   Snakes, see *Snakes*
   Spiders, see *Spiders*
Wolves, 192–194
Wood ticks, see *Ticks*
Wounds, see *First aid*

Y

Yukon, 17, 36, 79, 136, 145, 160, 175, 176, 186, 187, 192, 224, 238

Z

Zippo, 44

About the Author

Duane S. Radford is a native of Bellevue, Alberta and currently resides in Edmonton, Alberta.

He's an award-winning writer and photographer who started freelance writing and photography in 1995. As a member of the Bow Habitat Station Core Committee, Duane was bestowed an Alberta Order of the Bighorn Award, Alberta's foremost conservation award, in 1998.

He is a past President of the Outdoor Writers of Canada (OWC). He received the OWC highest award, the Pete McGillen Award, in 2017. He's currently a member of the Writers' Guild of Alberta.

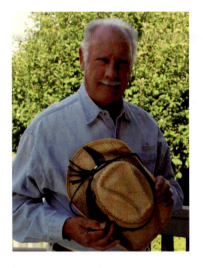

Duane is a member of the Alberta Fish & Game Association (AFGA) and represents this organization on the Antelope Creek Ranch Management Committee. He received the Henry Lembicz "Clean Air, Clean Land, Clean Water" award from the AFGA in 2016. In 2019, he received both the AFGA Fulton Award, its highest award, as well as the Canadian Wildlife Federation Roderick-Haig Brown Award, the latter for outstanding communications.

He retired as the director of Alberta's fisheries management branch. He worked as a regional director, regional fisheries biologist and fishery scientist for Alberta's Fish and Wildlife Division. He is certified as a Fisheries Scientist by the American Fisheries Society. He is an honorary member of the Great Plains Fishery Workers Association.

He has authored 950+ magazine articles and recipes in various magazines and newspapers in Canada and the United States, as well as eight books, five of which have received awards: *Fish & Wild Game Recipes* (2006); *Conservation, pride and passion: the Alberta Fish and Game Association*, 1908-2008 (2008), which he co-authored with Don Meredith; *The Cowboy Way* (2014); *The Canadian Cowboy Cookbook* (2014), co-authored by Jean Paré and Gregory Lepine; and *Fishing Northern Canada for Lake Trout, Grayling and Arctic Char* (2015), co-edited by Ross H. Shickler. He co-authored *Rodeo Roundup* with Wendy Pirk (2016) and authored *Canadian Fly Fishing: Hot Spots & Essentials* (2017). His eighth book, *Hunting Alberta*, was published in 2019 and made Edmonton's Capital City Press 2020 list of feature books.